'Clever, constructive recipes so that parents will be able to make simple, nutritious meals for their children ... We need more people like Jeanette ... well done, babe.'
Jamie Oliver

'Packed full of tasty, healthy and simple recipes using the best possible ingredients. Your children will thank you for buying it.'
Antony Worrall Thompson

'She's an inspiration to us – the more people who listen to her, the better the chances are of our children eating well.'
Hugh Fearnley-Whittingstall

'A dynamo, a true pioneer ... Every school cook and parent interested in food needs this book.'
Felicity Lawrence, author of *Not on the Label*

'Long before Jamie Oliver had even heard of turkey twizzlers, Jeanette Orrey was a school-dinners pioneer ... an inspiring book.'
Guardian

'She is living proof that one person who has a combination of energy and the right ideas at the right time can quite literally change the world. Jeanette Orrey is an inspiration.'
Patrick Holden, director of the Soil Association

'A fantastic, stimulating book from an inspirational woman.'
Lizzie Vann, founder of Organix Brands plc

'Jeanette started the movement to make school meals fun, tasty and healthy ... As a result, thousands of children are now eating healthier, tastier, fresher food for their school dinner ... We have a long way to go before all children are served the unprocessed, locally sourced and, where available, organic food that they have a right to expect, and that they need for healthy development. With Jeanette to inspire us, we will get there.'
Lord Peter Melchett, Soil Association

'One of my heroines.'
Jasper Conran

'I wish school dinners in my day had tasted as good as the meals dished up by Jeanette and her team ... By using locally produced meat, fruit and veg, Jeanette is giving local farmers and growers a fair crack of the whip.'
Lord Larry Whitty, Department for Environment, Food and Rural Affairs (Defra)

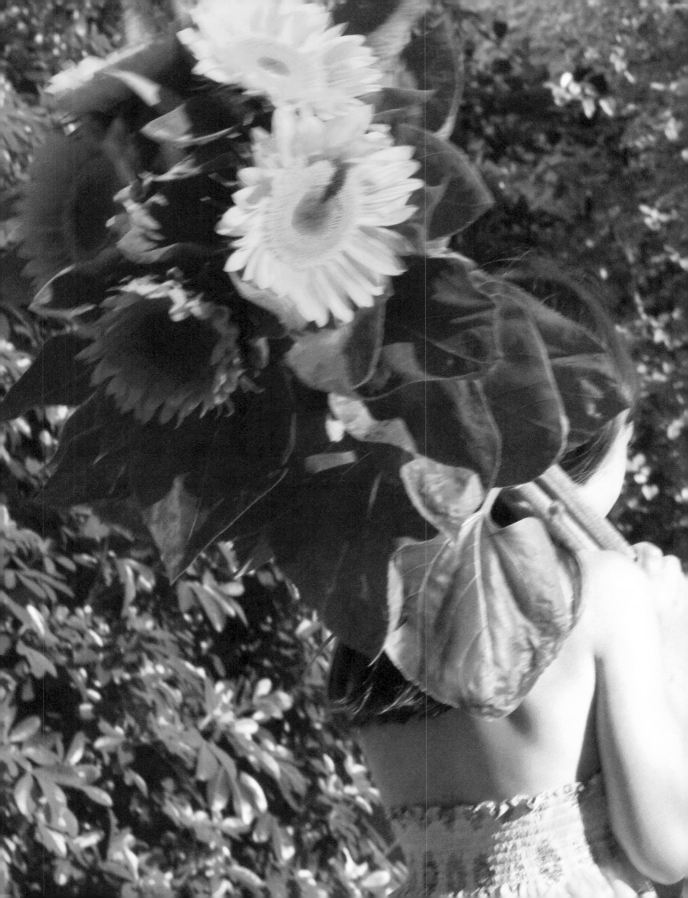

JEANETTE ORREY

WITH SUSAN FLEMING

SECOND HELPINGS
from THE DINNER LADY

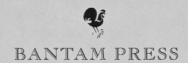

BANTAM PRESS

LONDON · TORONTO · SYDNEY · AUCKLAND · JOHANNESBURG

TRANSWORLD PUBLISHERS
61–63 Uxbridge Road, London W5 5SA
a division of The Random House Group Ltd

RANDOM HOUSE AUSTRALIA (PTY)LTD
20 Alfred Street, Milsons Point, Sydney,
New South Wales 2061, Australia

RANDOM HOUSE NEW ZEALAND LTD
18 Poland Road, Glenfield, Auckland 10, New Zealand

RANDOM HOUSE SOUTH AFRICA (PTY) LTD
Isle of Houghton, Corner of Boundary Road and
Carse O'Gowrie, Houghton 2198, South Africa

Published 2006 by Bantam Press
a division of Transworld Publishers

A catalogue record for this book is available from
the British Library.
ISBN 9780593054826 (from Jan 07)
ISBN 0593054822

DESIGN: Two Associates
RECIPE TESTER AND FOOD STYLIST: Caroline Marson

Typeset in Minion

Printed in Germany

1 3 5 7 9 10 8 6 4 2

Papers used by Transworld Publishers are natural, recyclable
products made from wood grown in sustainable forests. The
manufacturing processes conform to the environmental
regulations of the country of origin.

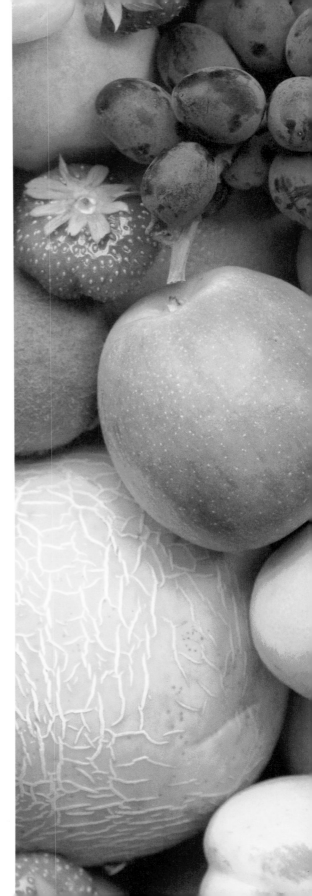

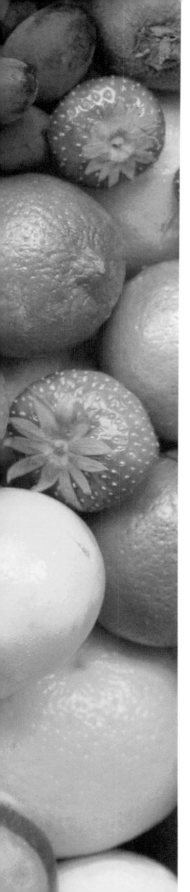

Contents

To my first grandson, Jacob James, and Susan's first granddaughter, Millie. Here's to the future generation.

Acknowledgements

Firstly I should like to thank my husband, George, for his continuing support and understanding of what I am trying to achieve, and for the thirty-two years we have spent together. My thanks too to my Mum and Dad, to Gareth, William and Jonathon, for looking after George while I was on my travels, and for keeping up with the laundry… And to my Mum-in-law, whom I now don't see nearly enough of.

I also owe a lot to David Maddison, head teacher at St Peter's Primary School (where all this began), and whom I go out to lunch with even now, time permitting. Thanks Dave, the next lunch is on you!

I should also like to take this opportunity to say a big thank you to the following :

To everyone at the Soil Association.

To my agent and friend Lizzy Kremer, to Susan Fleming, who has become a friend and who played a major part in the writing of this book. Special thanks to Diana Beaumont for her faith in me, Alison Barrow, Sally Gaminara, Katrina Whone, Lizzy Laczynska, Laura Gammell, Cora Kipling, Claire Ward, Alison Martin and everyone else at Transworld for making me feel at ease and for doing such a fantastic job yet again.

To Robin Matthews and Steve Baxter for the photographs. To Caroline Marson, who tested all the recipes, cooked and styled them for the photographs, and worked unstintingly on this book, and to Helen Crawley, nutritionist.

To Kevan Westbury at Two Associates and Phil Lord at Transworld for the wonderful design.

To Jamie Oliver for his continuing support.

To Hugh Fearnley-Whittingstall for his encouragement, and for the foreword.

To Jim and Bird Collins, Gary and Ali Stokes, Simon Owen and all the team at Ashlyns training kitchen.

To Eamonn Elliott and his team at the Devonshire Arms for looking after us so well.

To Innocent, who created a smoothie recipe for this book.

To the pupils of Forge Lane Primary School and all the other children who drew the fantastic illustrations.

Lastly, this book is for all the dinner ladies I have met – and am still meeting – on my travels the length and breadth of the country. Reach for the stars, ladies, you never know! I hope you enjoy this book.

6

Foreword

by Hugh Fearnley-Whittingstall

THE FIRST TIME I MET JEANETTE was at an organic food conference in Cornwall in the summer of 2004. I had heard a fair bit about her – and her school dinner revolution – but I was in no way prepared for the experience of hearing her talk. She took to the floor and simply told the story of the remarkable work she has done at St Peter's Primary School, Nottinghamshire, in transforming their lamentable school dinners into something sound, nutritious – and very tasty. It's a story only she can tell – and there are engaging reflections on it here, as well as in her fabulous first book, *The Dinner Lady*. And it is a story that, I believe, changes something inside everybody who hears it. It has certainly changed me.

Those of us who care about good food, and where it comes from, and believe that it is a vitally important part of a happy and healthy life, sometimes have a tough time keeping our spirits up. The size and power of the businesses and industries that grind our food culture into dull homogeneity and submissive mediocrity often seem overwhelming – unstoppable even. If, like me, you make a living in the world of food media, and hope, on the whole, to steer people towards a better relationship with food, it sometimes feels like a good day is one on which you are preaching to the converted, and a bad day is one on which you are fighting a lost cause.

Jeanette, who is one of the most remarkable people I have ever met, has bravely taught us that it really is worth reaching out to the unconverted – and that there is no such thing as a lost cause. For if ever a cause seemed lost in the world of food, it was surely the British school dinner. If ever a mission seemed doomed to failure, it was that of taking an absurdly low budget, an inadequately equipped catering kitchen and a thoroughly demoralized staff – not to mention a schoolful of kids weaned on to the dangerously addictive diet of highly adulterated processed food – and turning the whole thing round. Yet that is exactly what Jeanette did. And she has gone on to inspire others to do likewise.

Now the issue of school dinners, and their vital link to our children's health and happiness, is on the political agenda at a national level – and quite right too. And while Jeanette is quick to praise the fantastic work done by Jamie Oliver in raising the stakes and setting out the challenge for the coming years, she is too modest to mention that Jamie's campaign would have been more or less unthinkable without her mould-breaking groundwork that preceded it, and her continued input that accompanies it.

What I love about Jeanette is that she is not just a remarkable do-er, she is also a brilliant enabler – an inspiration to others to follow her example. And that's where her books come in. Anyone who knows a little of her story is likely to want to get on board in some way, and contribute to the success of her vision. But, of course, it's easy to

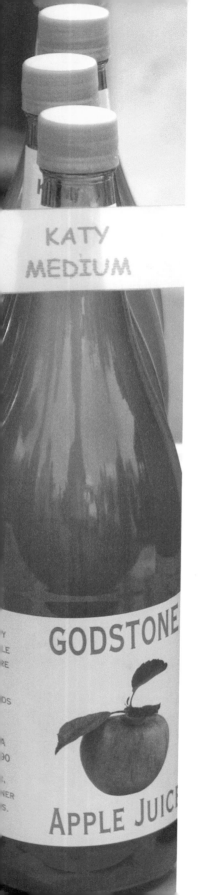

be floored by the very first question, 'where do I start?' This book, and its predecessor, *The Dinner Lady*, provide some very practical and welcome answers to that question.

Second Helpings is a book full of encouragement, reassurance and good ideas. Jeanette writes not just as a seasoned campaigner and good food evangelist. She writes as a mother and family cook. She knows that the way children are fed at home will be an even bigger influence on their future than the way they are fed at school. And she fully understands the pressures of time, and tight budgets, on the modern family household. Before we can re-enact a mini-version of her revolution in our own home kitchens, Jeanette asks us to reassess the way we think about, and acquire food. She encourages us not to be frightened of food 'in the raw', but to actively explore and enjoy it, so that the preparation of food for, and wherever possible, with, the family becomes a rewarding pleasure in itself.

Her tips for a sane and sensible approach to family eating are invaluable. For example, there is more digestible good sense in her four pages on 'Establishing good eating habits' (pages 89–98) than in whole books I have seen on the subject. Her recipes are sound and simple, even when they are exciting and adventurous: braised brisket of beef with barley (page 136) is a dish I would be equally proud to serve to my family, or to a table of paying diners at one of our River Cottage events – yet it is both economical and blissfully easy. And I am a particularly big fan of Jeanette's chapter on Breakfasts – because it recognizes not only the nutritional importance of a good start to the day, but the fantastic opportunity to get kids' creative food juices flowing every morning, by making breakfast fun and involving your children in preparing it themselves.

Above all, I find this is a nurturing and forgiving book, that will give its readers the strength and support to make real changes in the way they cook and eat. If you think you have got off to a less than ideal start on feeding your family, then *Second Helpings* offers you a second chance. And however well you think you are doing, there is, as Jeanette would be quick to remind us all, always room for improvement. I am proud to know Jeanette, and delighted to recommend this book, in the hope that thousands, if not millions, will benefit from her inspirational example, and indomitable good sense.

Introduction

WELCOME TO MY SECOND COOKERY BOOK. Since my first book was published at the beginning of 2005, I have had lots of letters and feedback from parents, teachers, dinner ladies and campaigners. All were in agreement that the answers to the problems of child obesity and poor health begin with the serving of good food at home and at school. The idea behind this second book is to provide dinner ladies and parents with even more good, tasty, child-friendly recipes. Some of these recipes are more adventurous than those in my last book, as they introduce different ingredients and tastes, although they are still easy to prepare. Simple and basic cookery is something I really passionately believe in, although you can only go one step at a time. I hope that you and your children enjoy this new collection of recipes.

If the letters I received show that there is a social 'heat' to food choices, there is also much evidence that the political heat is on as well. As far as school meals are concerned, Jamie Oliver has raised the stakes, and I for one thank him. He has done more in the school meals' campaign in less than a year than I believe anyone like me could have achieved in 15 years. He has echoed my own revolution, outlining the problems of poor-quality processed food, the cost-cutting, and the lamentable lack of knowledge in children (and sometimes their parents) of the nature of food and good eating.

Following on from Jamie's campaign, the Government has promised more money to schools, for more investment within the school kitchen for equipment, for more money to be spent on ingredients. This is very welcome, but will it be sustainable? We have been told we only have this for three years, but to my mind it is going to take a lot longer. It's not just about money for food on the plate; this is about food education, and that takes time. Head teachers and governors should not have to make a choice between books and food when balancing their budgets.

Many parents are demanding action on school meals, and some have taken steps themselves. I was very touched to receive a phone call telling me that a lady on the Isle of Wight was so impressed by my first book, *The Dinner Lady,* that she bought a copy for every school on the island. That was a positive reaction, but dinner ladies and campaigners still need your support as parents. The responsibility for food served to our children has to be shared.

My work has taken a different direction now and I am talking to and helping to train dinner ladies, rather than cooking myself. When I emerged from the insular world of St Peter's School, in a small village in Nottinghamshire, I wasn't properly aware of what was happening around the country, and did not realize how lucky I had been. On my recent travels (see below) I have seen that food poverty is still with us to a certain extent, and over the last few years I have learned a little about the history of school meals. The Liberal Government as long ago as 1906 recognized that adults were not achieving their full potential because of poor-quality – or too little – food during childhood. They passed measures to ensure that babies were registered with health professionals, introduced school medical examinations, and gave schools permission to give their pupils a meal in the middle of the day. This was the start of the school meal service, and an initial recognition of the absolute necessity of feeding the body to feed the mind.

Although we are 100 years on, sometimes it seems as though we have not progressed very far, for malnutrition is still with us. It's not the malnutrition suffered by starving children in Africa, the scarcity of food altogether – it's a lack of the nutrients that good food gives us. Our children – and often their parents before them – have been fed processed foods rich in sugars, fats and salt, and as a result we are experiencing epidemics of child obesity and diseases of adulthood in teenagers.

So what can we do? As concerned parents, teachers, head teachers, doctors, dinner ladies and, perhaps most importantly, town and county councillors and politicians, we have to try to change what has been happening. We have to persuade everyone that the food we buy, cook and eat should be of very much better quality. We have to persuade the food industry to change its stance: to become an industry that recognizes what people really need. Supermarkets say we are all time-poor, therefore ready meals and pre-prepared packets of cut vegetables fulfil our needs. But our real needs are much simpler: access to good fresh foods, the knowledge of how to cook them, and an enhanced ability to eat them with enjoyment. Supermarkets are at last making an effort, and recognizing that there is growing concern about where our food comes from, and are buying local food for local stores. This is a huge step in the right direction.

I want this book to reintroduce you to buying, cooking and eating well. I'm not a professional chef, politician or nutritionist. I'm a home cook, a school cook and a concerned human being. I want our food policy to change, I want 'food for life', I want to get to our children – to influence how they look at food and what they know about food. I want to enhance their appreciation of eating, by introducing them to new tastes, to bring them back from the extremes of junk and fast food to good home-cooked food. To do this, I have to reach parents, for they, along with schools, are the primary meal providers for most children.

The changed life of a dinner lady

When I wrote my first book I was working at St Peter's as a dinner lady, cooking fresh, local and organic food for the children's lunches. Well, that life has changed radically and I am now working for the Soil Association as School Meals Policy Advisor on our Food for Life project, and at Ashlyns Organic Farm where we have a training kitchen to enhance the skills of dinner ladies. It has been a very hectic year but my campaign for good food for children goes on.

My new responsibilities have taken me all over the country, meeting and talking to some lovely and sometimes famous people. The downside is that I have had to leave the kitchen at St Peter's after fourteen years.

Towards the end of 2004, I was still at St Peter's two days a week, and spent three days a week flying around the country for the Soil Association, advising schools on how to achieve Food for Life targets, and talking at conferences to parents, producers, head teachers and teachers, and government officials. In September I was in Essex, Wiltshire, Cornwall, Scotland, Hampshire, and a favourite place of mine, Abergavenny. October saw me in Middlesex, Newcastle, Aldershot and London. The London trip was daunting, as I spoke at the Guild of Food Writers' annual lecture dinner. I also had relations over from Australia – organic beef farmers – who wanted to see how the organic movement worked in the UK. I took them to see Bob Kennard in Wales and to Peter and Juliet Kindersley's farm, Sheepdrove, in Berkshire. By November I was in Scotland, Wales, Devon and London again. We also had a lot of TV and media interest at St Peter's as the school dinner issue began to grow. In December came the highlight of my year – a Christmas reception at Buckingham Palace in the presence of the Queen. I took my father with me, and he was so proud that at our family Christmas dinner he sat down with his Palace name-badge on (much to the amusement of the family)! The same month my husband George and I celebrated our thirtieth wedding anniversary and we spent a few days at the Devonshire Arms, Bolton Abbey, North Yorkshire. The saddest day of December was the 17th, when I cooked Christmas dinner for the children at St Peter's for the very last time.

January 2005 saw me at No. 10 Downing Street, and in Essex beginning to work on the plans for the new training kitchen at Ashlyns Organic Farm (see page 74). In February and March I visited five schools who were involved in Jamie Oliver's TV series *Jamie's Dinners*, and went to London for the Observer Food Awards (I had been a judge). Susan Fleming and I also spent some time in Norfolk writing this book.

April 2005 saw the publication of my first book, *The Dinner Lady*, with TV and radio interviews galore. Moving house at the same time was rather bad planning! In May I went to London, Kent, Essex, Swindon, Hampshire, Bristol, the Forest of Dean and to Bray in Berkshire, to Heston Blumenthal's The Fat Duck, for the *Daily Mail*. I also received an award from Glenfiddich, the 'Independent Free Spirit Award', which I shared with Jamie Oliver.

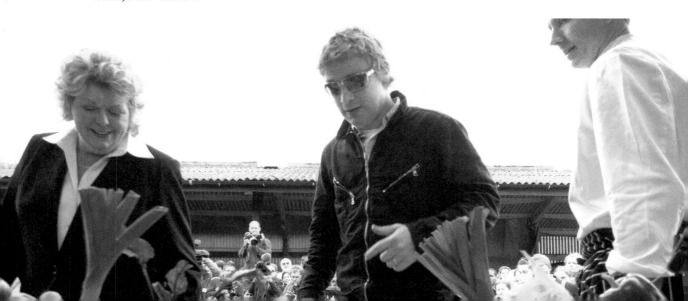

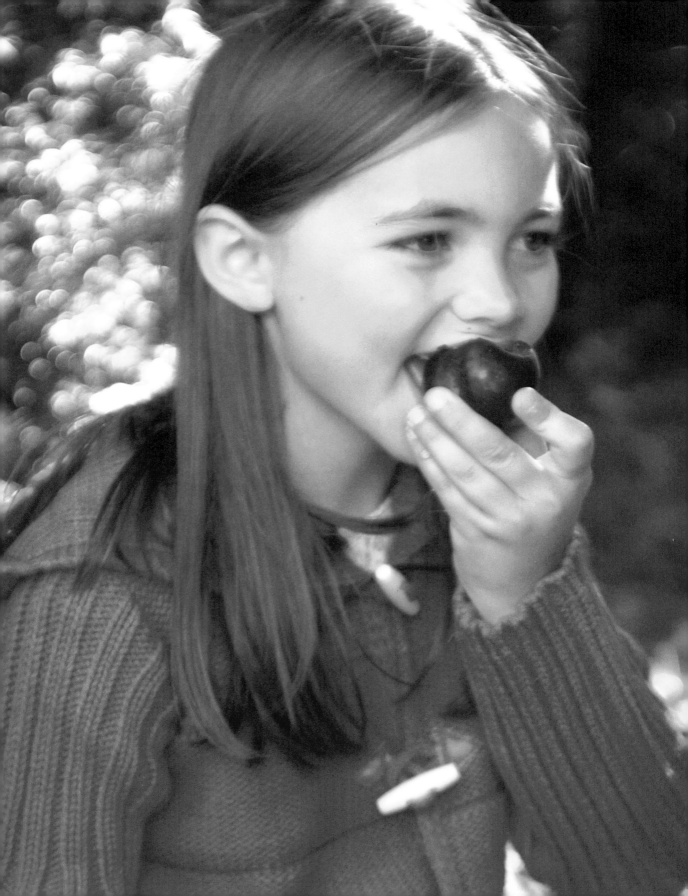

By June the training kitchen at Ashlyns was finished, and we managed, by the skin of our teeth, to hold a head teachers' conference the day after it was completed! Farm manager Gary Stokes and I were absolutely over the moon and for me at least a dream had come true. It wasn't until October that Jamie Oliver officially opened the kitchen, with over 300 guests and hordes of reporters and camera crews from here and abroad. In July we were joined by Simon Owen, a chef who worked on *Jamie's Dinners*, and he has been a tower of strength ever since. The rest of the summer was spent working at the training kitchen (three days) as well as at the Soil Association (two days), and writing with Susan, this time back at the Devonshire Arms. On 3 September 2005, our first grandson was born, a lovely little boy called Jacob James! Then there was more travelling, the Abergavenny Food Festival and, most importantly, photo shoots for this book.

In October, I was one of three judges for the Soil Association's Food for Life Awards. This year we were very lucky to get sponsorship from Highland Spring and *Body and Soul* (a *Times* supplement). We had over 100 entries (and a recipe from the overall Food for Life Award winner is included in this book, see page 279). In November, my travels took me even further afield, to Denmark, talking about our school meals. This was totally new to me, none more so than talking in English and listening to a conference spoken in Danish!

The future

The bigger picture is that we have to carry on the campaign for better school meals. This is a long-term investment in our future generations, and is something that I will continue for as long as I can. That's why I travel so widely meeting head teachers, cooks, governors, politicians and civil servants. And I am very pleased to have been appointed to the School Food Trust board, something that I believe carries huge responsibility. I hope I won't let anyone down, but we can all make a difference if we have a common goal. I should like to see school cooks and kitchen assistants given proper recognition, and the time and equipment to cook good fresh food. And, most importantly, I should like everyone to recognize what a very important job these people do, and how they are an integral part of a school. I shall carry on the fight, but you can do something too: talk to the catering staff in your child's school, and give them the support they deserve.

The crux of the matter is that we are all entrusted with the nation's most treasured possession – our children. Their future, our country's future, is our responsibility. I believe it is up to all of us to lobby for better food for our children, and I hope this book and its advice, recipes and stories will help you along some part of the way.

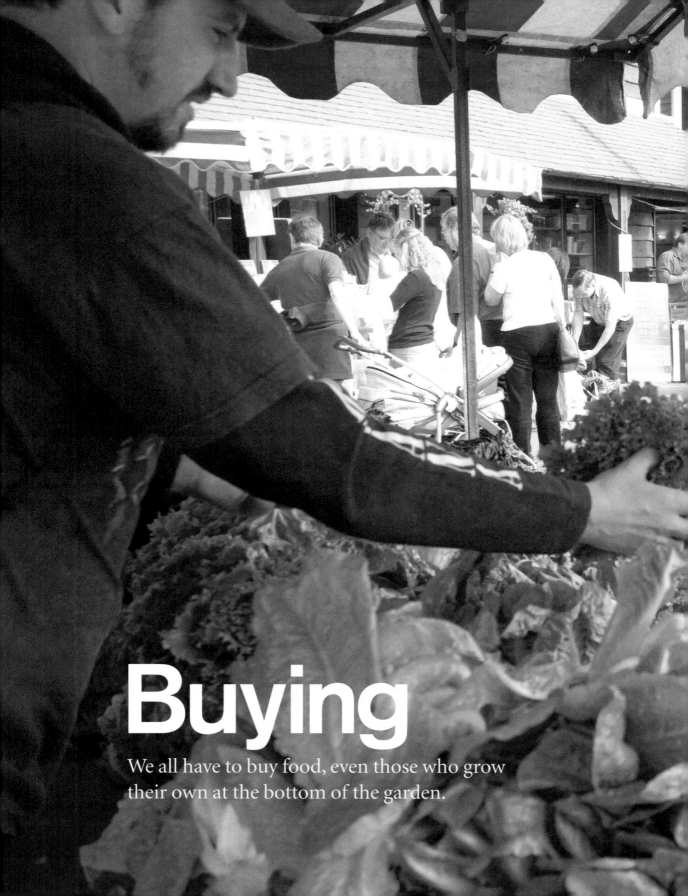

Buying

We all have to buy food, even those who grow
their own at the bottom of the garden.

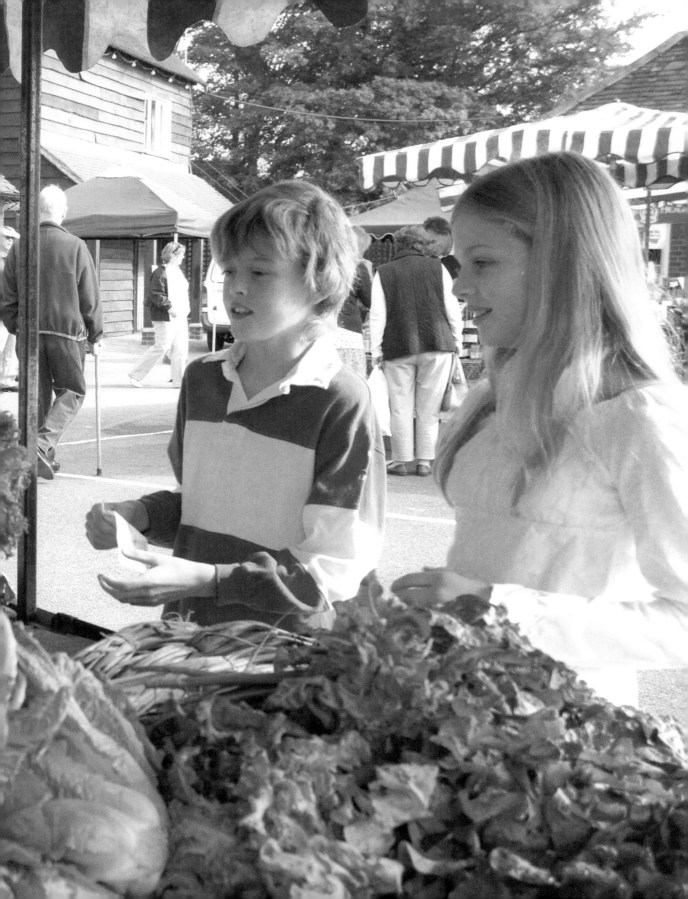

VERY FEW of us have the space or time necessary to grow enough wheat to make bread or pasta, or a field large enough to graze the cow that produces our milk and steaks. So, in the most simplistic terms, there is a production process: a farmer produces the fresh food, a middle man sells it, and then someone buys it. I'd much rather do without that middle man – the seller – and buy fresh food direct from the producer (I'll go into that later). But buying food should be a pleasure. It's all part and parcel of the greater picture: providing for our families, spending time with our families, and giving pleasure to our families.

No time to shop?

My life is so busy these days that I can't buy food in the way I once did, but how I did buy was the ideal. My Mum and Dad owned the village shop in Elston, and every day I would walk there pushing my son Gareth in the large Silver Cross pram that his proud grandparents had bought for us. I would buy my fruit and vegetables for the day, Dad bought his supplies from the local wholesale market three times a week, so everything was as fresh as you could get. I bought meat from the butcher opposite, which was run by a local farmer and his wife. (Both my parents' shop and the butcher have since disappeared.) For a young mother at home, this daily shopping was part of my social life. Because the village was so small, I would see other mothers from the playgroup, and we would stand and chat (if the kids had the patience). After my second son was born we got a car, and I would drive to Newark. There I would buy freshly baked bread and rolls from the baker, and something from the butcher, who sourced all his meat from nearby farms. Dad, my mother-in-law and I used to buy from the same butcher (it has also closed – it's now a dress shop).

While enjoyable, I have to admit that shopping did take time, and the word 'time' is important, as lack of it has had a great impact on how we all shop these days. We are said now to be a time-poor society, but why? Did we have more time years ago? The simple answer is yes, or at least women did, because they didn't go out to work (and they still do the bulk of the food buying). But since the 1960s, more and more women have been returning to work, full- or part-time, and they just don't have

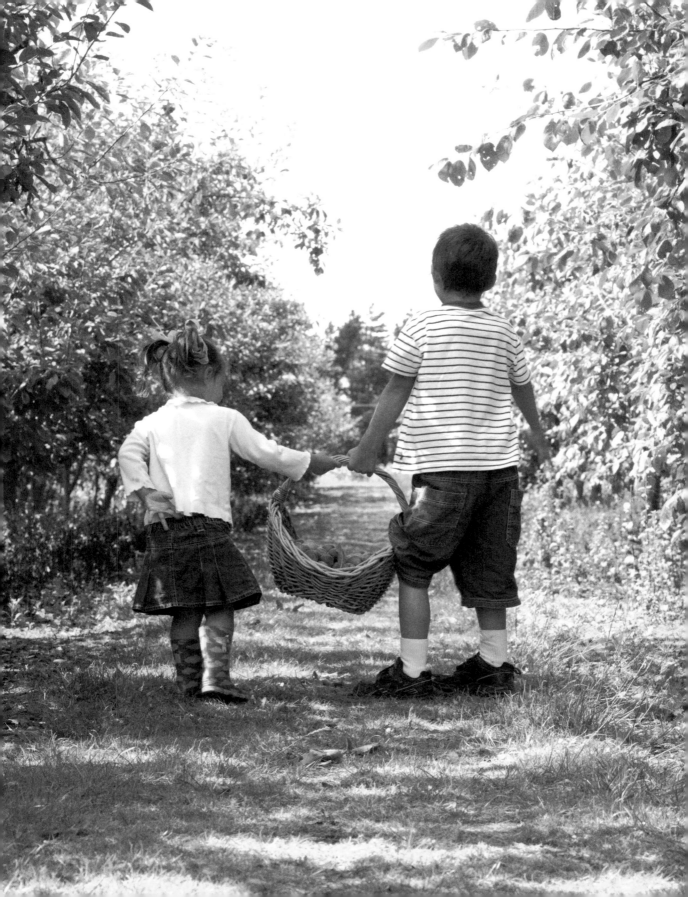

the time to shop every day (I'm a very clear case in point). Britain is now reputed to be the most hard-working country in Europe: British people spend more hours per week at the office, factory or shop – and travelling to and from that workplace – than any other nation, and this includes women. Because of this, we apparently have no time for what were the basics of life, such as buying food and cooking food. We do, however, allow ourselves time to eat – just – but what are we eating? We are buying food that has been designed to placate our supposed time poverty, food that has been pre-prepared, pre-cooked, modified, preserved, shaped, coloured and flavoured. This food does not make good eating, and the statistics on health and obesity – most alarmingly in children – relay their own message.

Buying food does take time and we have to allow for it. In the good old days we would buy fresh foods (vegetables, milk and bread) daily, and perhaps have a major weekend shop to buy the other household necessities such as cleaning products. Now we seem to buy all our food, even fresh foods, in one fell swoop – at the supermarket – once a week or, even worse, once a month. This shift in our shopping patterns has meant that the food we buy is now on the whole artificially preserved.

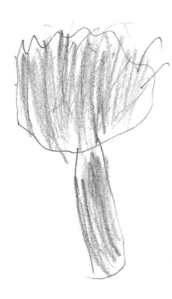

We are buying food that has been designed to placate our supposed time poverty.

For instance, when we bought bread daily it was made daily by the baker to be eaten straightaway. But since the 1960s, the Chorleywood bread process, a high-speed mechanical baking system, has been introduced. This uses flour 'improvers', softening agents and unhealthy hard fats, and the bread that is produced – the white sliced loaves available cheaply in supermarkets – now stays 'fresh' for days, which fits neatly into the current thinking that shopping should happen just once a week. This increased reliance on chemicals has also meant that convenience foods have become established in our buying lives.

It's a vicious circle: if we made time for it, we could buy fresh rather than modified and preserved food, we could buy it often and locally, and local shops would flourish. Thankfully, though, I believe this is at last beginning to happen. As I travel up and down the country, I have seen farm shops opening, farmers' markets flourishing, and consumers taking a genuine interest in where their food is coming from and how it is produced. Supermarkets are also beginning to listen. All this is having a very positive effect: by making time for shopping and buying, this generation is showing the next generation how to shop, and this has to be good for the future of real food.

SHOPPING TIPS
Planning can buy you time

● Use your supermarket for things you can't get locally, or the heavy goods like washing powder. Make a trip to the local shops for the rest, then freeze some.

● Make a list before going out, and stick to it. Impulse buying can be very wasteful if you can't use or freeze a fresh food straightaway.

● Stick a Post-it note on the fridge or notice board in the kitchen. Write on it things that are running low. *Check* it before going to the shops.

● Don't shop on an empty stomach, as this could lead to over-buying. This is particularly true when shopping with children: they are more likely to see something undesirable to eat and demand it if they are hungry.

● The best time to shop is just after breakfast: you won't be hungry, the stock will be at its broadest and freshest – and the shops are always quietest then!

● Think about those 'two for the price of one' offers in supermarkets. Is it really worth getting the extra one, or will the second one be wasted? And who will actually be paying for these offers? Ten to one it won't be the supermarket.

● Bulk buying of certain things can cause waste. They may cost less, but will they go off before you have the chance to use them? Flour, dried fruit and some cans can age and deteriorate in storage.

● Put all your fresh and frozen foods away as soon as possible. Move what is left in the fridge and freezer to the front, to use first (or throw away).

● Freeze basics such as fresh bread and butter: make sure they are wrapped properly, and then you will never be at a loss when the local shop is closed. You can freeze bacon well wrapped, and even milk, so long as it is in those plastic bottles.

● Buy fresh vegetables from the farm shop, blanch and freeze them in batches. Then you'll always have them when you need them.

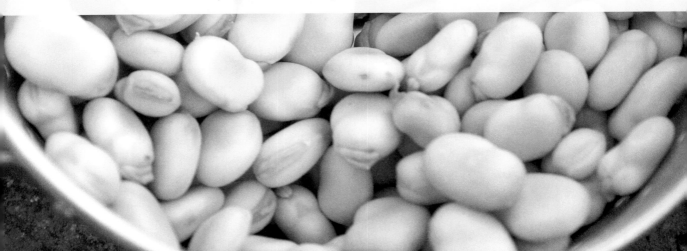

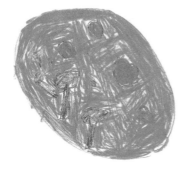

What price food?

There are so many books that explain better than I can what has happened in the last five decades. According to Felicity Lawrence, the campaigning journalist and author of Not on the Label, we now spend a much smaller proportion of our incomes on feeding ourselves than we once did. In the 1930s the average household spent 35 per cent of its income on food; today, the average is less than 10 per cent. True, since the 1930s we have become a wealthier nation, and people have become wealthier individually, but why are we spending less on our food? Is it because we are less interested in food and are eating less? Is it because food is more expensive and we can't afford to eat as much of it? Or is it because food is cheaper, and therefore we don't have to spend as much to buy what we need? I think it's the latter.

The cheap food culture

As our wages have risen, food prices have also fallen, because food has become big business. We all have to eat, and there's a profit to be made from that. Once it would have been simple: a cabbage would cost the farmer x pence to grow, he would sell it for y pence, say, to the local greengrocer, and the customer would buy it for z pence. The grower and seller would have made a profit, and the customer would have been happy. Nowadays, though, because of demand and competition, the picture is much less clear-cut.

Before the 1960s, small local shops and traditional Co-ops (the forerunners of the supermarkets, but established on much more egalitarian principles) dominated the food grocery market. This started to change when the first supermarkets began to appear in Britain (a concept imported from America). The supermarkets were fairly small at first, nothing like the giants they have become, and everyone thought they were a good thing (apart from owners of the local shops). Supermarkets offered a choice of foods – bakery, greengrocery, meat and fish, as well as packaged and canned foods, in theory everything you needed under one roof – and thus the idea of 'convenience' was introduced. The corner shop had once been 'convenient' because it was near, but now the supermarket took its place. It became more 'convenient' because, most significantly, supermarkets came to be seen as cheaper. The rot was setting in.

> We now spend a much smaller proportion of our incomes on feeding ourselves than we once did.

The supermarkets soon began to see how much influence they could have, and not just on their customers. They could influence the growers and producers too, and their requirements soon had farmers producing acres of a chosen vegetable specifically for them. The supermarkets could dictate price too, for they wanted to get the product as cheaply as possible, and sell it more cheaply than the local or corner shop. Prices paid to the farmer dropped as the supermarkets bulk-bought, and that price drop was passed on to the customer. Much later, the supermarkets started sourcing some vegetables and fruit abroad, where items could be grown at times when they weren't in season here. Some of these were items we could perfectly well grow in this country. Farmers abroad could produce the food needed even more cheaply (see Fairtrade, page 30), and thus the farmers here were faced with what has become known as globalization, yet another layer of competition and stress.

With all this happening, we inevitably started to become used to the concept of cheaper food. We now expect meat, for instance, to be affordable on a daily basis, whereas it was probably a once-weekly treat for our grandparents. But why should food be so cheap?

Cost at the expense of quality

When millions needed feeding after the food shortages of the Second World War, the Government demanded high productivity from the farmers. As a result, the old system of mixed farming (where a farmer breeds a variety of animals and rotates his crops every year) was gradually replaced by intensive agriculture, whereby a farmer concentrates on a single product – what is known as monoculture. Specialization inevitably increases yield, and farmers were also given subsidies by the Government, depending on the quantities of food they produced. (Subsidies may help the farmer in the short term, but they devalue the true cost of what he produces.) Gradually, greater quantities of food were produced, and prices became cheaper.

But that cheaper price comes at a cost. You only have to drive through Lincolnshire today to see vegetables being grown in huge fields with very few hedgerows. This is one example of monoculture or, to put it another way, our disappearing heritage. In addition, where the rotation of crops once naturally disrupted the life cycle of single-crop pests, now the fields have to be sprayed with pesticides. To boost the fertility of the land and crop (previously achieved naturally), artificial fertilizers are also used. The same applies to intensively reared farm animals: pigs, cattle and poultry were not long ago routinely given antibiotics, growth hormones and fertility-boosting drugs. These chemicals are now known

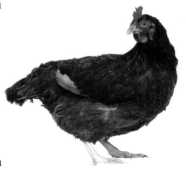

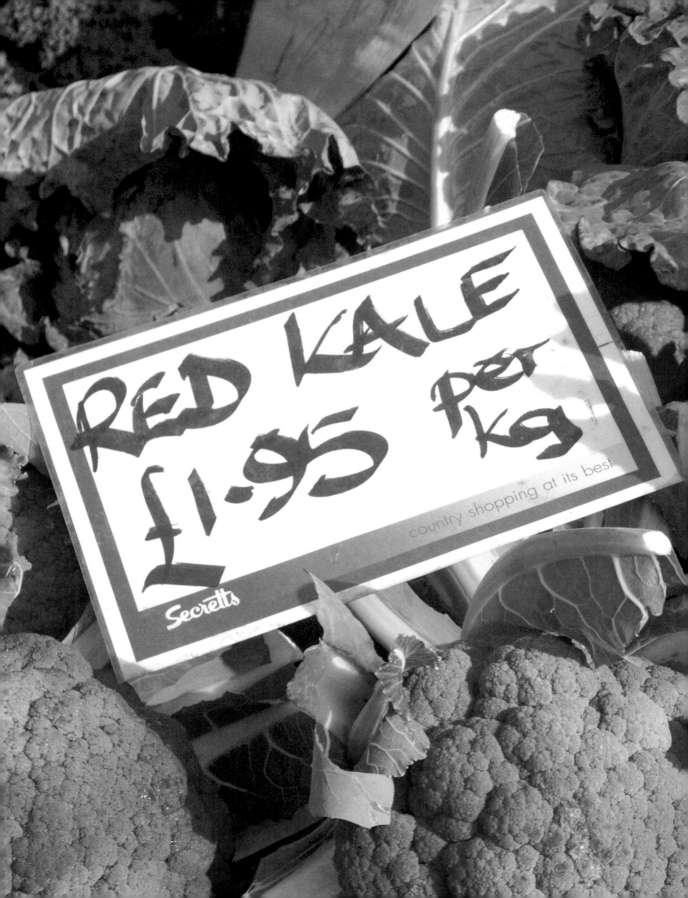

to cause damage to the soil, to ecosystems, to wildlife and indeed to humans – for residues can still be found in the food that we buy and eat. (They also 'cost' us in a different way, for the run-off of pesticides and fertilizers into the water system requires millions of pounds in purification before we can drink it.)

And, of course, the intensification of agriculture has led to a huge diminishment in animal welfare. Where once animals used to roam around outside – cows and pigs in their fields, poultry in the farmyard – now the majority are kept inside, all in the interests of high yields and low cost. We have all seen television documentaries about battery chickens and crated veal calves, and have heard about the diseases caused by intensive rearing, among them bovine spongiform encephalopathy (BSE), Creutzfeld-Jacob Disease (CJD), avian flu, E. coli and campylobacter outbreaks.

All this has made me passionate about knowing where my food comes from, and how it has been fed or cultivated. And indeed it was partly this concept of cost at the expense of quality that led us to opt out of Council control at St Peter's.

As a dinner lady, I wanted my children to be fed the best possible ingredients, although I was always constrained by budget to a certain extent. Now, when I am talking at conferences, I always ask, 'How much do you pay for a cup of coffee?' The answer is usually in the region of £1.50 to £2. If this is acceptable, how then can people expect school caterers to feed children a two-course lunch for an average of £1.50? Food should not be considered a 'cheap' part of our daily lives. It's not an 'expense', it's a necessity, and what we eat is what we are.

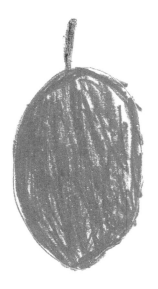

What should you buy?

The ideal is to buy fresh food, locally produced and in season, and, ideally, organically produced. That might seem like a lot to ask, but if we all did this we would soon loosen the stranglehold the big food conglomerates have on our supplies of food, there would be less food available to go to the convenience food manufacturers (this market grew, apparently, by 400 per cent in the 1990s), small shops would flourish, and our farmers, local or organic, would be able to make a decent living again.

Fresh food

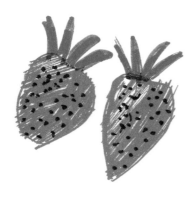

Vegetables are not fresh if they have been sent from one country to another, or even from one end of one country to the other. Fruit is not fresh if it has been picked under-ripe then been shipped from abroad (although we have no choice if it can't be grown in this country). Meat is not necessarily fresh if it has been jointed, rinsed and wrapped in polythene and clingfilm. The same goes for fish. Fish is actually a difficult one, because I think we all have problems with fresh supplies unless we're lucky enough to live near a fishing port. (But even then, in some places I've heard that most of the fresh catch is sent straight to the French, Italians and Spaniards, who are willing to pay a proper price for fresh food.) Fish is often frozen at sea as soon as it is caught, though, so it can be as good as fresh when you get it (and see page 30).

Fresh vegetables and fruit are packed full of nutrients (vitamins and minerals): the longer they take to get to you, the more these nutrients will have diminished. Fresh does not necessarily mean a shining clean potato or an unblemished tomato. Potatoes covered with a light coating of soil will probably be fresher than those washed for cosmetic purposes. And some of the tastiest tomatoes I have ever eaten have been misshapen, with blotches on them, and streaks of green and yellow through the red. A Channel 4 programme, Dispatches, actually took some of our home-grown tomatoes to Spain. Spanish housewives said they wouldn't buy them because they had no taste. And ironically, the Spanish are growing some varieties of tomatoes especially for the British market, tomatoes they wouldn't buy or eat themselves because of that same lack of taste! And that's one of the major points. Quite simply fresh meat, fish, vegetables, and fruit do taste better than food ripened in storage, and why should we buy a food for any other reason than good flavour?

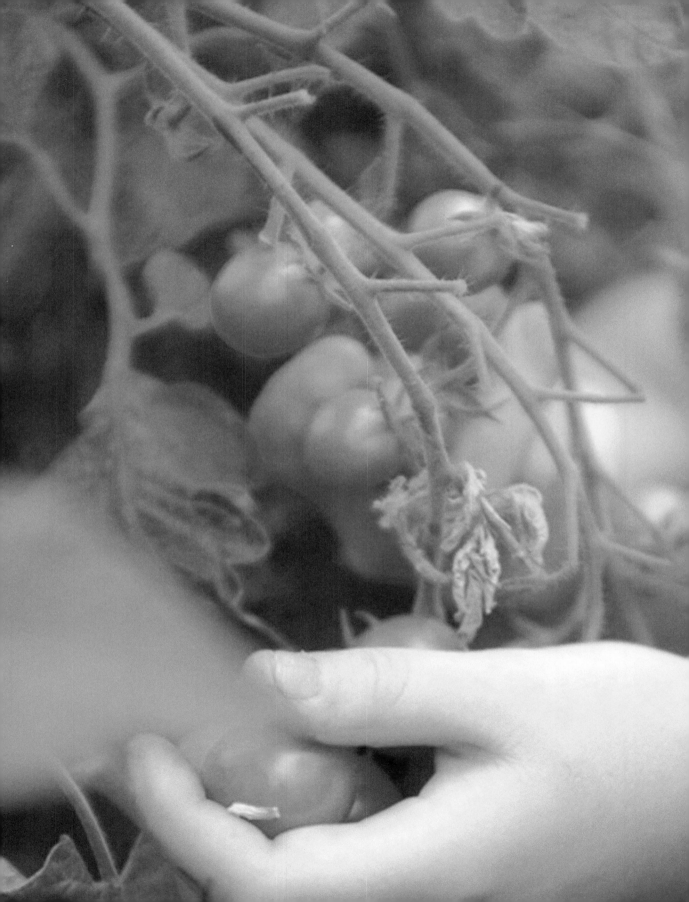

Caff

Ringden Farm
East Sussex

rich flavour. Crisp and juicy,
aromatic crunching apple. Can
be eaten throughout winter.
It is recommended.

Ashmead's Kernel

Grown By Ringden Farm
Flimwell, East Sussex

A high quality, old dessert apple with a sweet,
slightly acid, highly aromatic flavour. With very firm,
crisp, juicy flesh and russetted green/red/yellow
skin. It is picked in mid October and ready to eat in
November onwards. It was raised in Gloucester by
Dr. Ashmead in about 1700.

Red Pip

Local food

If you live in the country or a small town and can buy from local suppliers, freshness is virtually guaranteed. Vegetables and fruit will not have made marathon journeys to get to you. And if you buy local apples, say, you might be instrumental in keeping an orchard, and a less common variety of apple, in existence. If you're buying meat or fish locally, you might be able to get to know your butcher or fishmonger, and you can ask him where his products come from, and how they were fed and raised. I did this when I began the changeover at St Peter's, and I learned a huge amount. I still ask in shops and especially in restaurants – sometimes to my husband's embarrassment – if they know where their produce comes from. (I am very careful about where I shop now, and will only eat in restaurants that I trust.) It is not so easy in big cities, but it is possible.

Buying local foods means fewer food miles (the distance travelled in producing and distributing food), which means fewer emissions from delivery vehicles and less traffic on our already overcrowded roads. Maybe this is a little simplistic, but to my mind, every little helps. Animals bred and slaughtered locally will not be transported long distances, which can stress them. There will be less packaging too – a brown paper bag is all that's required. And as a bonus, local foods mean local farms, which children from local schools can visit, to see where their food comes from.

Most importantly, if you're buying locally, you're helping the local economy. High-street shops often employ local people who may be able to walk to work, reducing traffic even more. You can probably walk to the local shops too, thereby saving on petrol and petrol emissions, and you'll get a little exercise as well! If you give your money to a local shopkeeper or farmer, he will probably give his money in turn to another local person (staff) or business (supplier), so the money will stay in the community. This makes that money, by a mathematical concept called LM3 (Local Multiplier 3), worth much more. Joanna Blythman, in her book Shopped, says that every £10 spent locally is worth £25 to the local economy. That same £10 spent at the supermarket is only worth £14 to the local community (for most of it goes out of the area, usually to shareholders).

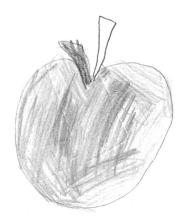

Seasonal food

You wouldn't think it, looking at the produce available in supermarkets, but food seasons do still exist. Green leaves start appearing in spring once the weather starts to warm up, new potatoes and asparagus appear in May–June, strawberries in early summer (along with imported seasonal peaches), and apples, pears and blackberries are around in the autumn. Foods and tastes associated with a particular time of the year used to be part of our annual eating pleasure, but that has all changed. Globalization means that foods can be flown in from anywhere at any time of the year, so that seasonal savour has gone.

Up until recently there were at least two generations who were unaware of the natural growing cycles of this country. When I was at school, we used to have what we all called 'double-digging', which was an hour's lesson when we used to plant vegetables and salad leaves, learn about the seasons, and later on enjoy taking the produce home. Unfortunately, this seems now to have been taken over by IT, information technology, and slowly over the years we seem to be losing this natural part of our education. People now blithely accept that strawberries (all one variety, see page 42) can be bought all year round, flown in from Spain, the USA, Israel …

The same two generations will also be unaware of the flavour of home-grown, fresh, local, seasonal foods, something that really worries me: as food becomes blander or less essential in flavour, our palates are changing. With less appreciation of flavour, will we become less interested in real food and turn increasingly to convenience foods? This was beginning to happen, I believe, but now a slow change seems to be taking place all over the country. A lot of primary schools I have visited have their own fruit and vegetable patches, and this food that the children have grown is being sold to the school kitchen to be used in the children's school lunches. What better way for them to taste and enjoy the flavour of home-grown produce?

Organic food

Organic foods are grown or reared without the aid of artificial chemicals, so are the antithesis of intensive agriculture. Until about six years ago I didn't know very much about organics. Now I work part-time as School Meals Policy Advisor for the Soil Association – the principal organic certifying body in this country! In the last few years the sales of organic foods have multiplied: the UK market is now the third largest in the world, after the USA and Germany. Most supermarkets have organic sections (Sainsbury's were in the vanguard of the whole organic sales impetus), and there are even chains of specifically organic supermarkets (Fresh and Wild and Planet Organic, to name but two). It was also recently announced that the department store Barkers, in Kensington, London, is to become the flagship store of an American organic organization. So you should be able to buy organic foods quite easily.

Growing or rearing foods organically takes longer and the yield tends to be lower – because no chemical fertilizers or growth hormones are used – so they are more expensive than 'conventional' foods. But I think our food prices are too low anyway. There is an ongoing debate about whether organic foods are better in flavour or healthier than non-organic. I believe that they are. Research shows that organic fruit and vegetables contain less water, possibly making them tastier. In the Journal of Alternative and Complementary Medicine, it was reported that organic crops contained up to 27 per cent more Vitamin C, 29 per cent more magnesium and 22 per cent more iron than non-organic crops. A British Medical Association report found that some pesticide residues in non-organic produce are linked to cancer, Parkinson's disease, foetal abnormalities and a decrease in male fertility. Organic eggs have up to twenty times more Omega-3 polyunsaturated fatty acids (see page 80) than factory-farmed ones; and organic milk has higher levels of Omega-6 fatty acids, which have been shown to help prevent cancer. Quite apart from that, I would be happy to pay more in the knowledge that the foods were produced in a sustainable way, one that is beneficial to the environment. I believe we have to value our food.

Having said that, many people still worry about organics. Standards of certifying bodies around the world do vary, and what the Soil Association would not pass as organic, another might. Over 60 per cent of organic food sold in the UK is imported, which also raises the question of food miles. When the ethical farming group Sustain analysed a sample basket of 26 imported items, it found that they had travelled some 150,000 miles. If they had been air-freighted (using aviation fuel), they would have polluted the atmosphere with the same amount of carbon dioxide as a four-bedroom household cooking meals for eight months. The continuing involvement of big food conglomerates in organics vexes me as well: they are still in the market to make profits, and they could apply the same pressures on organic suppliers for high yield and a cheap supply chain. That could lead to cut corners and to a diminishment in quality… a familiar story.

My advice is to buy your fresh organic food locally and seasonally, from farm shops, farmers' markets, or get involved in a box scheme (see page 40). Concentrate on home-grown organic produce, or if you buy imported food, choose something that has travelled least far – perhaps buying Italian rather than New Zealand kiwi fruit. It has been said that each kiwi fruit flown from the southern hemisphere consumes its own weight in aviation fuel. That doesn't sound like sense or sustainability to me… However, due to climate change, it's now possible to grow kiwi fruit in Kent and Dorset. It's all topsy-turvy!

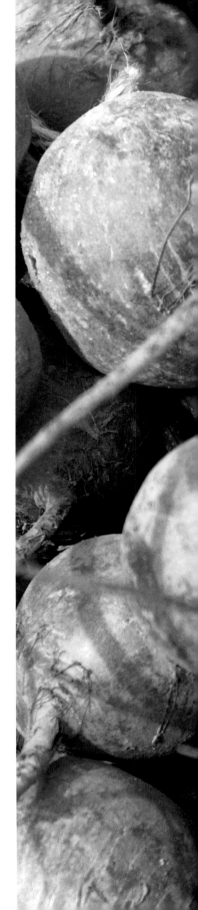

Fairtrade products

These are products from around the world that are protected by an organization called the Fairtrade Foundation, set up in 1994. There are many links between organics and Fairtrade, but the latter focuses more on the workers' conditions. Fairtrade assures producers and workers a 'fair trade', good working conditions (safety, no forced child labour, fair wages), as well as a fair return on the costs of production. Fairtrade is moving more towards organic production, with protection of the environment and an ever-decreasing usage of artificial chemicals. Your concerns about food air miles can perhaps be balanced by the fact that the growers of bananas in the Dominican Republic, say, are protected. (Farmers in this country could do with a bit of 'fair trade' too, if you ask me.)

The pupils at St Peter's are learning about Fairtrade in the classroom, and in the kitchen more Fairtrade products are being used, so the children can link what they are learning with what they are eating. So, if you do see Fairtrade foods (and drinks, plants, flowers and some fabrics), do buy them. You may pay a little more, as you do with organic foods, but you are positively helping people in less wealthy parts of the world to help themselves. I would rather Fairtrade than aid.

Frozen or chilled foods

Much frozen food is very good indeed. Often it is 'fresher' than anything you buy in your local shop: for instance peas grown for Bird's Eye are picked, podded, packed and frozen within 12 hours – much less time than it might take fresh peas in their pods to reach your local greengrocer. The Food Standards Agency (FSA) has recently confirmed that frozen broccoli, peas, cauliflower, sweetcorn and carrots contain higher levels of vitamins than imported fresh equivalents. And frozen fish is what a lot of us have to rely on: much fish is filleted and frozen at sea, so is almost as good as fresh. However, it has been reported that after reaching these shores and the British suppliers, it can be defrosted, packaged and sold as fresh – as many chilled prawns, shrimps and crayfish are. Packaging doesn't necessarily tell you all this, so you have to be careful. A clue might be the label that tells you not to freeze (because it has been frozen once already).

What you could be confused by is the chilled produce you can now find in many supermarkets. A chilled hamburger or fishcake has become 'fresher' in our minds than frozen. But beware: to keep it 'fresh', the chilled product can be packed with additives, many more than in the frozen equivalent. Chilled vegetables and salad leaves come ready cut –

to save you time – but nutrients are lost from vegetables once picked, then again from the cut surfaces, so what you are doing is further reducing nutrients you hoped to get. Go for the frozen peas in preference to the packets of podded ones in the chiller cabinet. In addition the packets will probably also have been filled with 'modified air' (not declared on the packet), which slows down the natural process of decay. Research carried out by Which? magazine found that sliced chilled runner beans in packets contained nearly 90 per cent less Vitamin C than fresh beans.

Genetically modified foods

Genetic modification or GM is the artificial transference of genes from one organism into the DNA, or biological make-up, of another, quite unrelated species. The transferred gene in the new genetically modified organism will serve a particular purpose (making a plant insect-resistant, delaying a fruit or vegetable's ripening) or add nutrients (such as Vitamin A to rice). The main GM foods grown worldwide at the moment are maize (corn), soya beans and oilseed rape. We have fought to keep this country free of GM foods, but it may be a losing battle, and the health of our children is what is at stake.

Profit is once again behind the use of GM. Four multinational agrochemical companies control the GM market. They claim that this biotechnology is all for the benefit of mankind – alleviating world hunger, eradicating weaknesses in crops, making crops more nutritious, creating crops that can be grown on poor land. It may all sound very positive, but these companies could take over the entire 'global larder': through patents they could control the supply of seeds, the farmers and their land (if they didn't own it already), what is grown and how.

Many people have been against GM from the start. The trouble is that no-one is entirely sure what potential health hazards these mutated foods might hold. The other concern is that of cross-contamination: pollen from GM crops would inevitably spread to non-GM crops, and conventional farming – let alone organic farming – would be virtually at an end.

For political and health reasons I avoid GM foods (Greenpeace have an excellent guide to GM-free buying; see their website). Some 80 per cent of processed foods contain maize or soya, which might be GM, so it's easy to avoid processed foods. Many foods that we buy every day – like bread, butter substitutes, cereals, even some baby foods – may not ostensibly contain GM ingredients, but no manufacturers can guarantee that milk or eggs in their products are not from animals that have been fed on GM feed.

CHILDREN AND SHOPPING

Most parents, especially mothers, don't have much choice when it comes to the combination of children and shopping: they have to take the child/children with them. As is well known, this can be at best boring for the child, and at worst a battle to the death over something he or she has seen and wants. (If you dread the thought, you can buy on-line.) Very young children won't be interested in shopping, but from about the age of five, perhaps when they have begun to help you in the kitchen, you can involve them. The trick is to make it fun for them – and you might find that you educate them in the process. As I always say, food can be allied to maths, geography, history and a host of other subjects. I think teaching children how to choose good ingredients and involving them in the buying of food is just as important as their learning to cook.

I prefer to take children to smaller local shops, markets or farmers' markets, as there is more potential friendliness and human contact, which they love. At a farm shop, they might meet the cow that supplies their milk, and see that peas come in pods from a plant, not out of a packet from the freezer. Butchers may not be so popular, but a fishmonger's can fascinate children – there might even be a live crab! (When our children were little, we always holidayed in Wells-next-the-Sea, Norfolk. William, my middle son, adores fresh fish, especially crab. Once we got up at the crack of dawn so that he could choose a crab off the fishing boats. The woman at the local fishmonger cooked it for him and even now, though he is over six foot tall and 21 years old, she still remembers and recognizes him.) If the shop is a delicatessen, cheese shop or baker's, children may be able to taste samples. Visiting several smaller shops or wandering round a market is probably more interesting too for a child than being wheeled in a trolley up and down brightly lit supermarket aisles and being told, 'Don't touch!' But they can also enjoy the supermarket, if you fine-tune your buying strategy.

Work out a menu with the children before you go. Give them a few choices – pasta, risotto or cottage pie, say – and then let them help you select the ingredients. If you're making a tomato sauce for pasta, you could get them to pick out some tomatoes and onions; if cooking a mushroom risotto, they could pick out so many medium-sized mushrooms with long stalks. Even children of under five can choose vegetables or fruit on the basis of colour – one red and one yellow, for instance. It will take time, I admit, and some stallholders might not respond well to small hands on their produce. But if you then let them help you prepare the food when you get home – wiping the mushrooms, halving the tomatoes – they may be more inclined to eat the dish in which they have been so involved. You can lavish praise on them too, for choosing and helping to make such a successful meal.

By allowing children to participate in the selection of fresh foods from as early a stage as possible, they may be less inclined to hanker after foods they see advertised on the TV. But if you engage them early enough in the basics of good food and nutrition – 'Sugar is not good for any of us, and that cereal or fruit yoghurt has loads of sugar in it' – then you can even make a game out of reading labels on child-orientated packets or jars they might crave. A slightly older child could well be horrified by the listings of ingredients, half of which are patently not 'food'. It's potentially a huge subject, but . . .

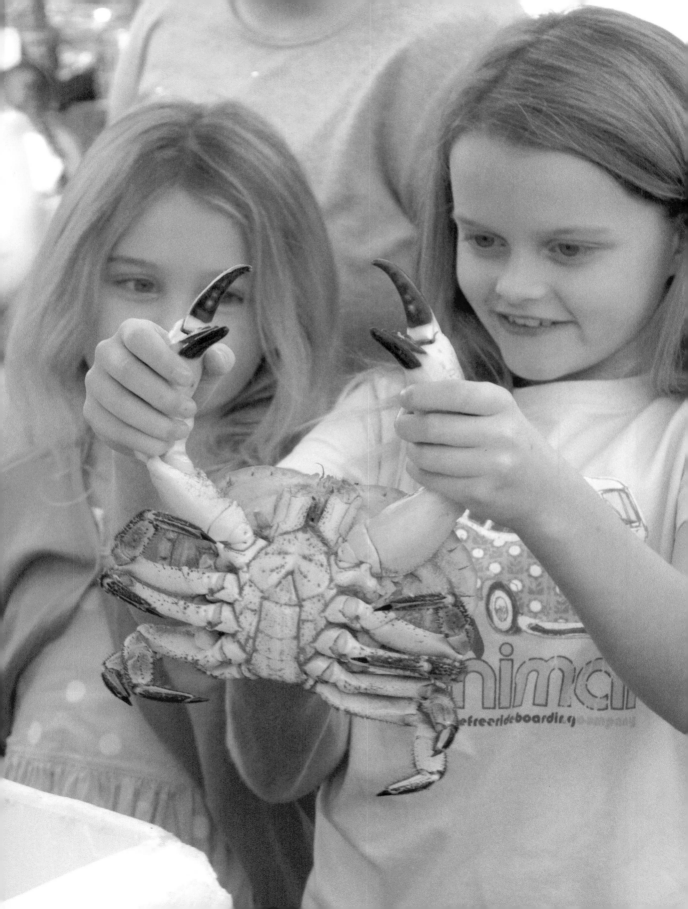

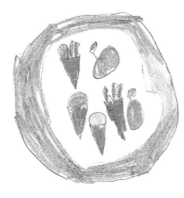

Where to buy?

Where and how you shop for your family depends to a certain extent on whether you live in a city, town or village. In towns and cities you have to rely on local shops or supermarkets – or, if you're lucky, you can buy at farmers' markets, which are becoming increasingly popular. In the country you have much more choice, but that is possibly too simple a statement: with local village and high-street shops closing due to the ever-encroaching supermarkets, sometimes there could be less choice.

Local shops and markets

We all used to buy our food in local shops and markets, wherever we lived, as I did at my parents' shop. Mum and Dad ran their shop for 38 years and it was part of the village social life, but it had to close because of competition from the supermarkets in Newark. But now, after a gap of seven years, Elston has opened a 'community shop', run by paid and volunteer staff, in a Portakabin near the village hall. Maybe people are beginning to realize what a vital part a village shop can play in village life after all.

In the 1950s small shops and Co-ops held 80 per cent of the food market. Now the situation has virtually reversed, and it is supermarkets who control 80 per cent of the fresh fruit and vegetable market, with local shops disappearing fast. Apparently, between 1995 and 2000 – in only five years – we lost one-fifth of our local shops and services. It seems extraordinary to me that this should have happened, but there is an inevitability about it, as Joanna Blythman reports in her book, Shopped. Basically, if a supermarket opens on the edge of a town, some residents will use it and some will still shop in town, but the people who had to come into town to shop will no longer do so. The result is that enough revenue is lost by the town centre that the high-street shops close anyway, so everyone has to use the supermarket and the centre inevitably dies.

But where would you rather shop? I prefer to buy my meat from Mr Smith, the local butcher, and know where it has come from, and how it has been produced. Mr Smith will probably have tips on how to store it, prepare it, cook economically with it, what to serve with it. However, most important of all, I think, is the opportunity for a chat. This to me is what buying should be about: it's an excursion with a decided purpose, but it can and should be relaxing. And what could ever be considered relaxing about the supermarket!

I do urge you to use local food suppliers. If everyone did it, small shops could flourish once again.

Farm shops and pick-your-own

In the country you have access to farms and farm shops. Farms once commonly sold goods directly to consumers, but have become so enormous, catering for 'agribusiness', that in the last decade or so you'd have been hard put to find anything resembling a traditional farmyard! The tide is turning, though, and small to medium-size farmers – often by choice, sometimes from necessity – are starting again to sell food grown, produced or made on the farm, directly at the 'farm gate'. The 'shop' itself may be a stall in the farmyard or literally at the gate, or it may be a converted barn or dairy. Some farmers get together to form co-operatives to sell their produce at a centralized venue.

According to the National Farmers' Retail and Markets Association (FARMA), there are currently about 3,500 farm shops in the UK. These shops offer foods (fruit and vegetables, dairy or meat and meat products) produced either on the farm itself or locally, and some of these foods are organic. So freshness and seasonality – two of my favourite words – are to the fore. Many of them sell other goods too: they often have home-baked cakes and breads, home-cooked frozen foods, ice-creams and yoghurts, local cheeses, fruit and herb teas, fruit juices, wines, cider (and mead), organic flour, jams and preserves, honey and honey mustards (as well as

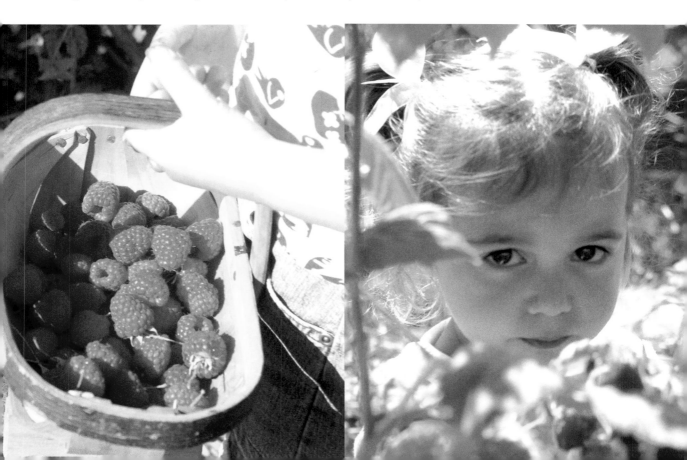

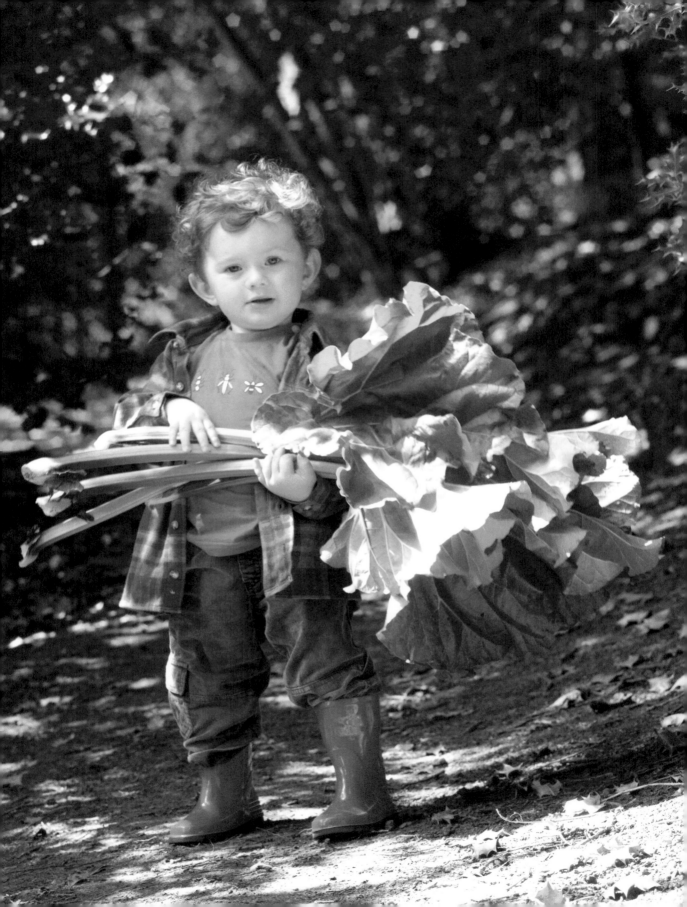

beeswax skin creams, candles and polish). There's even a farm shop at Chatsworth House, established by the Duchess of Devonshire, which sells its own beef, lamb and venison (from the park). In the course of 2004, they sold 25 tonnes of home-made sausages and in December of that same year they sold 25,000 home-made mince pies! One year I got my Christmas turkey from Chatsworth, an organic Bronze, which was delicious (although my father said he still preferred his cockerel). I must admit that I'm a sucker for many of the secondary products at farm shops.

Again according to FARMA, some 1,000 farms nationwide offer a pick-your-own service (including the Queen's Sandringham estate in Norfolk). Pick-your-own offers the ultimate in freshness and seasonality, and children love it. It was a favourite outing for my boys in the summer. We've picked raspberries, strawberries, blackberries, blackcurrants and peas, and at some farms you can even cut your own asparagus. What most appeals to me about this concept, so far as children are concerned, is that it connects them directly to their food, to where and how it is produced. Not only are they touching and smelling, they can be tasting as they go along too, thereby using all their senses at once and discovering wonderful, truly fresh flavours. (Although, if they overindulge, as William did once on blackberries, the pleasure could later turn to stomach-ache.)

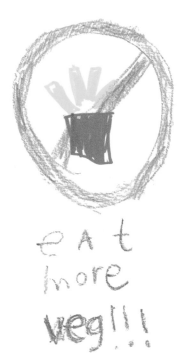

eat more veg!!!

By buying from farm shops, you will be getting truly fresh produce, and you will be directly helping the local farmers and the local economy. You'll also be helping in an ecological sense too, because you'll be avoiding all that supermarket packaging – you might get a brown paper bag if you're lucky… And if you live locally, you'll be cutting out all those food miles as well.

Farmers' markets

The first farmers' market in England opened in Bath in 1997 and since then some 450 others have been established (a process which suffered a huge setback when the countryside was struck by BSE and foot and mouth). The movement had been long established in America – a 1995 survey of 772 American farmers' markets suggested that more than 25,000 farmers sold only at farmers' markets – and indeed it was an American, Nina Planck, who masterminded many of the London markets.

It seems amazing to me that the concept of a 'farmers' market' is so 'new' in this country. People all over the Continent have always bought their fresh food from markets, and we used to do it ourselves until not so long ago. The basic idea is that farmers who are 'local' – this can vary in certain circumstances – sell their own fresh produce direct to consumers. The National Association of Farmers' Markets lays down several criteria:

Buying

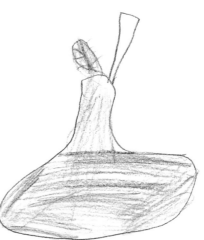

- The food must be locally produced.

- The principal producer must attend the stall.

- All 'primary' produce must have been grown, reared or caught by the stallholder within the defined local area.

- All 'secondary' produce must have been brewed, pickled, baked, smoked or processed by the stallholder, with at least one ingredient originating from the defined local area.

'Local' is usually defined as within a radius of 30–40 miles of the market, but in the case of a huge urban sprawl such as London, or in very remote rural areas, 'local' can stretch up to 100 miles. In London, producers are permitted from within 100 miles of the city-circular M25 motorway.

Produce is much the same as that sold in farm shops. My local market sells fruit, vegetables, salad leaves, juices, cheeses, herbs, meat (raw and processed/cooked), fish, eggs and breads. I must admit, though, that I have seen produce on sale occasionally that looks like it has come rather further than it should, and I do wonder how stringently the 'rules' are being applied. A friend of mine went to a farmers' market with a market inspector, and saw a stallholder selling lettuce from boxes marked 'Spain'. The inspector had a quiet word, and said if it happened again, the stallholder would be off the market. These safeguards are reassuring, because we don't want farmers' markets to go the same way as some car boot sales. However, all you have to do is ask a direct question of the stallholder – and I'm never shy of asking questions!

I think the idea of farmers' markets is wonderful, and I know that many of my London friends couldn't do without them. (At least they are no longer at the mercy of the supermarkets, now that so many local shops have closed.) Apart from being able to buy fresh food, there are benefits to the producers. Smaller farmers can remain more viable, and indeed stay in business, because they are growing what people want – and the local economy is boosted. Many more unusual and diverse crops can be grown, which adds to the consumers' and growers' pleasure, and to a diversity in nature. All the environmentally unfriendly issues are avoided: no airfreighting and air miles, no over-packaging, no processing, no preservatives or additives.

Children love going to markets, and it's another way of keeping them in touch with how and when their food is grown, and what it looks like. (Jamie Oliver's horror when the kids at a school in Durham didn't

THE BEST SAUSAGES I HAVE EVER TASTED!!

ALL HAND MADE, CONTAINING NOTHING BUT BEST ORGANIC PORK (OURS!) LOVE, CARE & ATTENTION.

HOME MADE DRY CURE BACON GAMMONS, S.

PROPER ORGANIC EGGS FROM OUR SMALL FLOCK OF FREE RANGE HENS

WONDERFUL FRESH VEG, NOT SPRAYED OR TREATED WITH ANYTHING AT ALL, TRULY 'HOLEY'

AND ALL FROM LEAFY SURREY — REAL LOCAL FOOD, ALL GROWN ON OUR FARM

WWW.LEEHOUSEFARM.CO.UK

Food is like petrol, for your body. Fruit has sugar, but a special type of sugar! A sugar that is very unusual!

by Rachel Hartigan, age, 8

recognize any of the foods he showed them will remain with me for ever!) Visiting a market is enjoyable for everyone. Many people who go to farmers' markets have said that it's the social aspect they like best: they can actually talk to the suppliers and growers about their produce, meet neighbours and friends – usually at a designated time per week. In London, I know that markets have brought back a sense of community to many neighbourhoods. Even HRH the Prince of Wales has been quoted as saying that a farmers' market '… will foster greater understanding between town and country by helping to reconnect people to the land'.

So if there is one near you, go and have a look, and have a good day out. Don't forget, though, that they are very seasonal, so don't expect the same choice of fruit in November as you might have had in July. And don't be put off by the weather: even if it's pouring with rain, the stallholders will be there – it's their living, after all – and they need your support.

Box schemes

The Soil Association was instrumental in introducing the idea of box schemes into the UK in 1992, and there are now over 500 schemes, some 350 of them certified organic. A farmer or farm shop delivers a weekly box of fresh, locally grown, seasonal, possibly organic produce to your door or a drop-off point such as an office or your child's school. Some boxes include imported organic produce, especially during what is called the 'hungry gap' in late spring. Many boxes include a recipe card telling you how to cook a certain vegetable or a whole dish. Some organic meat boxes are also available now countrywide, which means that a few lucky customers don't have to dash around the supermarkets at the weekend.

Schools can actually benefit from a box scheme financially. Among others, Abel & Cole, a London-based firm, runs a venture whereby organic vegetable boxes are delivered to London schools, paid for in advance by parents, from which the school gets a percentage.

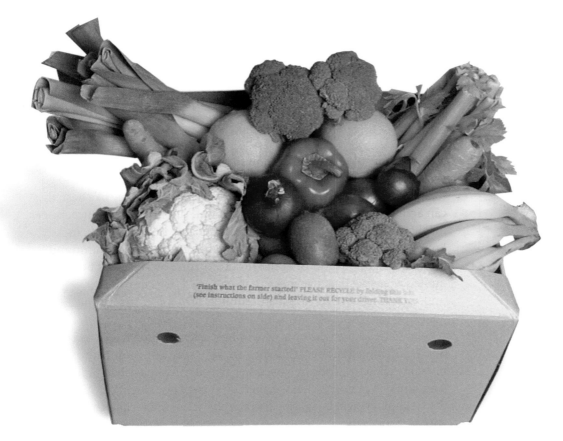

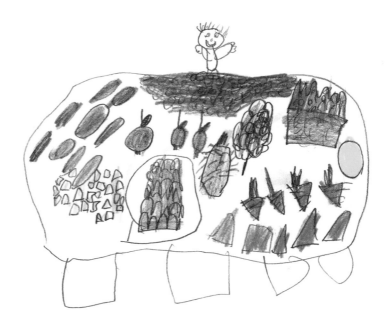

Supermarkets

Nowadays we do all – or at least most (80 per cent is the statistic) – of our food buying in supermarkets. It's a vicious circle: as supermarkets spread, their convenience and cheaper prices wean us away from local shops, and the local shops begin to close, reducing the shopping options. Food is undeniably big business, and supermarkets and agribusinesses are now amongst the largest and most powerful conglomerates in the world. But profit usually means corners have to be cut and belts have to be tightened. In any other business this might be acceptable, but in food it's definitely not, and leads to the use of pesticides, growth promoters, additives, etc. Profit may be good for the shareholders, but it is not good for the consumer, the producer or the environment.

Supermarkets are convenient as they appear to offer a huge variety of foods at reduced prices, and they are undoubtedly here to stay. But there are disadvantages. For a start, those apparently endless aisles actually offer less choice. Strawberries are a case in point. Britain has always grown strawberries, and we know that English strawberries at Wimbledon time are unbeatable. Well, they used to be. Now one variety, the Elsanta, is being grown to the exclusion of many others. Why? Because supermarkets know that it stores and travels well.

The vegetable and fruit shelves may look gleaming and inviting, but when we know we should be eating the very freshest of foods, are the supermarkets offering us them? Possibly not. Supermarket chains are now so centralized that a runner bean from Dorset will probably have travelled up to a depot in Northumberland and returned to the south of England before it reaches the shelf. (Some 40 per cent of haulage on our roads is food-related.) And even when a supermarket claims that the food is local, in reality, according to a Friends of the Earth survey, 'local' in supermarket speak means only that it has been grown in the UK. And an amazing one-sixth of what we pay for food in the UK goes on the cost of the packaging.

Supermarkets are responsible for reducing the value of food. They compete against one another to lower prices, and although the consumers may benefit financially, the producers don't. Farmers' prices are forced down by the buying power of the supermarkets, so much so that often they are obliged to sell at less than cost. In addition, supermarkets insist that customers want perfect vegetables and fruit – cauliflowers with leaves just so (even though we don't usually eat them), potatoes gleaming, carrots with not a wisp of root. This is madness. Vegetables just do have blemishes, and a little bit of soil (they are grown in it, after all). But supermarkets tend to reject produce that does not conform to their requirements, leaving the farmers to find an alternative market, at the last minute; or worse, the food is rejected and can be used as landfill. A study commissioned by Biffa, Britain's leading waste and recycling company, found that of the 5 million tons of fruit and vegetables supplied to Britain's supermarkets each year, one-fifth is lost in the packing, grading and preparation processes. Although some of the 25–40 per cent of foods rejected by supermarkets is resold to the catering trade or food-processing companies, or used as animal feed, surely there must a better way? I can think of one for a start – they could be used within the school meals service.

But why on earth do we now seem to be shopping with our eyes? Cosmetically perfect food does not taste better. We should be shopping 'by mouth' – seeking flavour, not appearance – and indeed the essential flavour of vegetables and fruit is often lost these days because things are so intensively grown, have travelled so far (often from abroad) or are simply not as fresh as they might be.

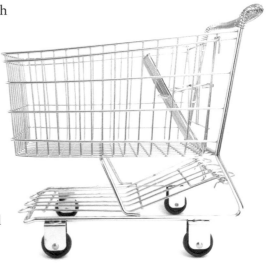

There is good news though. Supermarkets are beginning to listen to consumers. You can buy organic food (choose food that has not travelled too far), and they are stocking more and more Fairtrade products. Some supermarket chains are consciously selecting local fruit and vegetable varieties. If we continue to ask, they will supply.

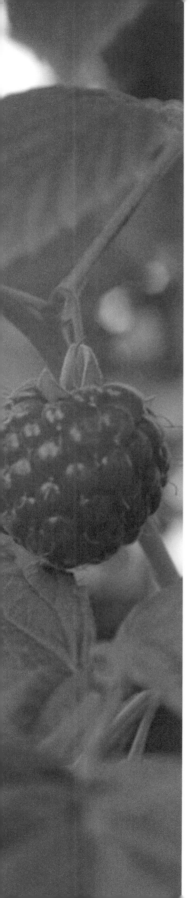

Or grow your own

I'm not the one you should look to for instructions about growing fruit or vegetables at home – that should be my Dad or my husband. If I see a worm, I'm off! But it's a distinct and positive thought if you have the space. You could also rent an allotment, something that has seen a huge take-up again. Or, at the very least, you could grow some herbs on a sunny windowsill. Buying seeds from a good supplier isn't difficult, although preparing a vegetable bed, sowing, watering and waiting for the fruits of your labour will take time . . . but it's fun.

By growing your own, you will be getting the best of all worlds – fresh, local (you couldn't get more local!), seasonal and organic (because hopefully you won't be applying chemicals). You and your family will experience the taste of fresh vegetables straight from the ground, and you will also feel very proud of yourself. Perhaps the most important aspect of growing your own involves the children. They can help, and it's a great way to get them engaged with the food they eat: I bet that any previously picky vegetable eater will be more enthusiastic about a lettuce, carrot, bean or radish that he or she has grown.

Many schools have their own vegetable gardens in which the children can work as part of the curriculum, and they can eat the results at lunchtime. It was Alice Waters, renowned chef/proprietor of Chez Panisse in Berkeley, California, who initiated the idea, with what she called The Edible Schoolyard. At her local junior school, the pupil-tended garden has become the model for a growing international trend: there are now over 800 schools across the UK doing the same. These are backed by various organizations such as Garden Organic (previously HDRA Henry Doubleday Research Association), Duchy Originals (the Prince of Wales's food company), and Adopt-a-School (run by the Academy of Culinary Arts, the professional chefs' guild). These educational and edible gardens teach science, nutrition, history and geography, as well as address the obesity problem. In both America and here, parents have reported that their children come home enthusing about things previously ignored – like cabbage – and completely change their attitude to fresh foods. That sounds like a good idea to me.

St Peter's has its own vegetable patch, and the new catering manager, Sarah Plumb, along with a parent and the children, is busy sowing and planting vegetables to have in their school lunches. Again, the whole-school approach.

ADVERTISING AND CHILDREN

When you're out shopping, the 'pester power' of children can be daunting. 'Can I have that?' 'Why not?' And then there might be a scene: we've all seen it, an embarrassed parent and a tearful child. The same thing can happen at home, and it's all to do with television. There are few homes without a TV set these days, and few children who don't watch children's programmes for at least an hour a day. To have them quiet and rapt in front of a favourite cartoon character allows you to unwind or prepare their supper. But those programmes are interspersed with advertising, mostly for food products (our British screens carry the most child-orientated food advertising in Europe). If that advertising were for fresh greens or fruit, I wouldn't mind, but most of it is for highly sugared cereals, cakes, biscuits or confectionery, most of which is highly processed 'junk food'. If the likes of David Beckham advertised carrots, there would be a shortage!

But it's not just on TV that advertising entices our children. Food packaging is specifically designed to attract them, using bright colours, jazzy graphics and those self-same cartoon characters they like so much. And packets of cereals, say, often offer gifts, which are another persuasive pester-power factor. Worst of all are the cynical campaigns run by some companies to persuade schoolchildren to buy foods that will lead to some reward for the school – new sports equipment, for instance, if they collect enough empty wrappers, packets or cans.

Encourage your children to be part of a good food culture. Tell them which foods are full of sugar, and explain why they are not for them. If your children are used to fresh, home-cooked food, the occasional tasting of these sugary foods might surprise them – they could be *too* sweet, too salty or indeed too bland. But don't make this into a treat. And always remember that you are the one, not the child, who wields the buying power; you are the one holding the purse-strings.

There's one small word that I feel isn't used often enough, and that's 'No'.

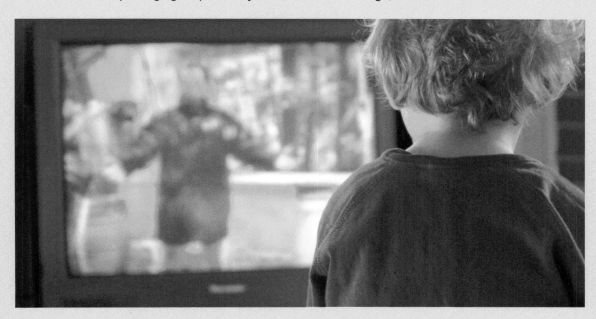

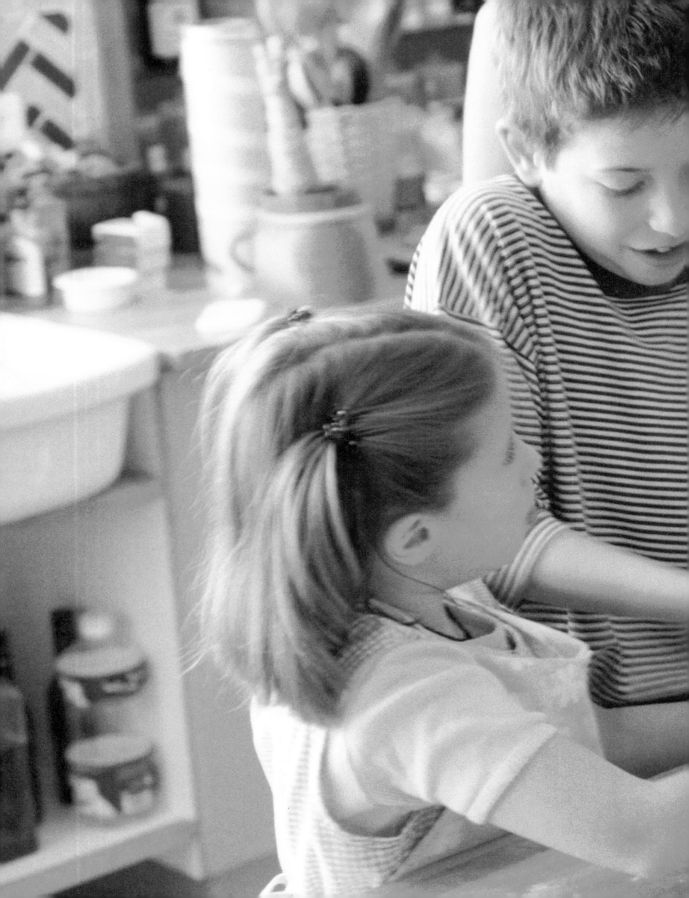

Cooking

We should all be able to cook. It's a basic life skill, and one of the pleasures of life.

MY MUM and Gran taught me how to cook – although if you read my first book, in which I admitted to cooking fish fingers and chips for my new husband's first meal at home, you wouldn't have thought so! Now that so many families are fragmented across the country and cookery is no longer taught in schools, we have lost the idea of passing cookery skills from generation to generation. We have also lost to a great extent the feeling that good home cooking can bring people together. We even seem to have lost our taste for good food. All this has happened only in the last 40–50 years or so – in just two generations.

According to research commissioned by the food manufacturer Dolmio, mothers spent about 13 hours a week preparing meals in the 1950s, but by 2005 this had fallen to 5.9 hours. Alarmingly, this means an average of 13 minutes per meal. To my mind, the only thing you can do in 13 minutes is pop a ready meal into the microwave. Mintel, a market research organization, also published a report on changes in the way we eat. They interviewed 25,000 people: most respondents said the change was the result of the pressures of modern life and the changing position of women in the family and home. As with food buying, women do most of the food preparation, and as more women went out to work, they became 'time-poor', so instead of cooking, began to rely on alternatives. Hands up the food industry, who stepped in with a multitude of packets to which you just add water; ready-prepared meals to heat up in the microwave; and chilled, prepared ingredients (salad bags and chopped vegetables for example). The reliance on these instant foods could be one factor in the rising levels of obesity and ill-health in the general public and, most disturbingly, in children. It was the reliance of school-meal providers on prepared and pre-cooked foods that led to my own personal revolution, and to the many revelations in Jamie Oliver's television programmes about school dinners.

For our own health and well-being, and that of our children, we need to eat *fresh* foods, and it is important that we know how to cook them. I would like to see good home cooking the norm in every household, and every school canteen.

Cooking is *not* heating up...

They say that we watch more TV cookery programmes in the UK than any other nation in the world, and own an enormous amount of cookery books – but we still can't cook! I say instead of watching that cookery programme, get into the kitchen and cook. But that's not what we are doing. We have become a nation of food 'watchers' and food 'heaters'. The recent report from Mintel found that the British now spend an unbelievable £18 billion on supermarket ready meals, 63 per cent more than in 1994. I find that horrifying.

TV dinners and other convenience foods

It all began in 1953–4 when a salesman, Gerald Thomas, from a frozen-food company in Nebraska, invented the first ready meal. The company had hundreds of tons of unsold turkeys after a disappointing Thanksgiving, and needed to get rid of them. He adapted the airline foil tray idea, designing his own version with three sections: one for meat, one for vegetables, and the other potato. A turkey dinner was the first offering, and it was an enormous success. Television was fairly new then, and in one fell swoop the ready meal, marketed as a 'TV dinner', took over, and family eating in the United States was never the same again.

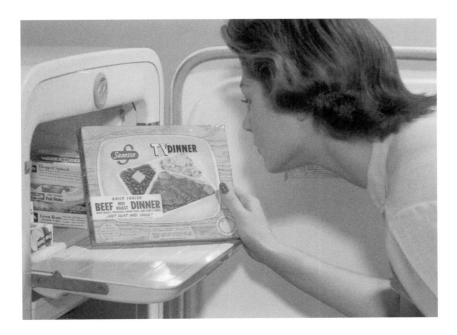

Here in Britain we were slower to adopt the idea. Bird's Eye and Findus were selling frozen fish and vegetables from the 1960s, but the TV dinner didn't arrive until the 1970s. In the 1980s, the decade when the number of women working boomed, we took to it with a vengeance. Sales of microwave ovens peaked: they were the perfect answer to the demand for getting food on the table fast. And 'fast food' took on a new meaning thereafter, with fried chicken and burger takeaways (in the most famous burger company, their avowed aim is to get you in and out as fast as possible, with the toy of the moment, although they too are adapting).

Is domestic cookery dead?

I hope not, and I am fighting hard to keep it alive and kicking. But it's difficult when ready meals are so easy to obtain. The reliance on factory-produced, rather than home-produced, food has been reflected in other ways as well. Houses are built with kitchens that are often too small for a dining table – and of course there is no dining room. Where, then, are people meant to sit and eat? In front of the television, I presume, with their 'TV dinners' on their knees. I know someone who has four children, who doesn't even own a cooker: she heats everything in the microwave, and has done so for about 20 years. And, of course, if she doesn't cook properly, how are her children expected to learn to cook?

> Houses are built with kitchens that are often too small for a dining table. Where, then, are people meant to sit and eat?

And they are not the only ones. A friend of my son William came back from his first term at university recently looking and feeling dreadful. We got chatting, and it turned out he was living on fast food because he didn't know how to cook. It was also costing him a fortune. I suggested he might cook himself a baked potato, but even that very simple process was a mystery to him. How many more kids are like that? They're not just lacking essential life skills, they are endangering their health through eating the wrong things. If this generation of children – boys *and* girls – don't learn how to cook and eat properly at home, then we have to teach them how to do so at school. Domestic cookery is a cornerstone of family life and I hope the brief notes following might help you return happily and successfully to the kitchen.

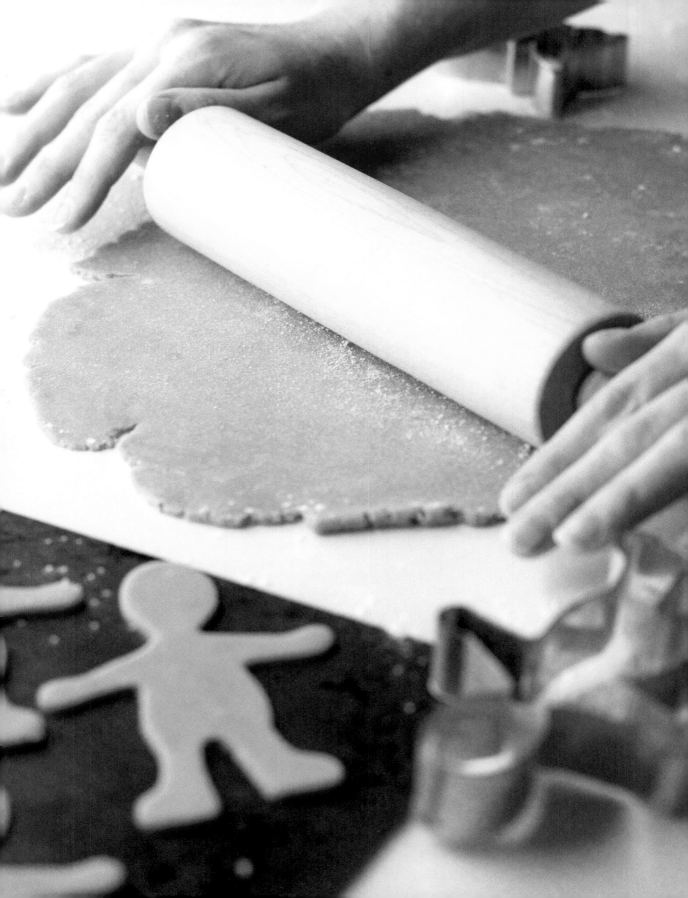

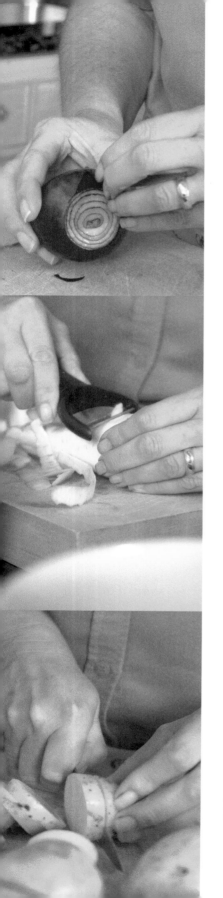

Top up your techniques

Many of you will be familiar with some or all of the techniques here, but quite a number of young people are obviously not. You shouldn't have to be a chef to be aware of at least three cooking methods, perhaps boiling, roasting and frying. I'm not a chef, just a home and school cook who is passionate about food, but by going to some cookery classes I learned a few additional cookery skills. Some cooking methods are essentially healthier, simpler or safer than others, and in most situations the less healthy method (frying for example) can be replaced by an alternative (grilling or baking). The healthiest cooking techniques use little or no fat. And remember that the fresher the food is, and the less 'messed around', the more nutrients it will retain. For it's a sad truth that more than half of the nutrients of any food you eat will have been destroyed before it reaches your plate, depending on how long since it was harvested, how you store and prepare it, and on how you cook it.

The following are just a few ideas that might help you cook more enthusiastically, more simply and more healthily.

Preparing your food

● Wash all food before cooking it. Remove the outside leaves of lettuces and cabbage, which are often a bit tired anyway. I wipe mushrooms rather than wash them (they retain some of the liquid used to wash them). If you must, peel vegetables and fruit minimally, as most of the nutrients are near to the skin.

● Cut up vegetables at the very last moment, and cook them as 'whole' as possible, for as soon as any large amount of surface area inside a plant is exposed to oxygen, the nutrients (vitamins and minerals) are quickly lost. For preference, cook a cauliflower or broccoli head whole, and then break into florets. Slice or blend other vegetables after cooking.

Boiling/simmering/poaching

In this country, we boil eggs, we boil beef and bacon, we boil potatoes and green vegetables – the latter to death, some say, though less so these days.

● **Boiling** means cooking in a lot of liquid over a high heat.

● **Simmering** is when the heat is turned down so that the liquid has only slight surface movement.

● **Poaching** is when the heat is turned down even lower so the water is hardly moving.

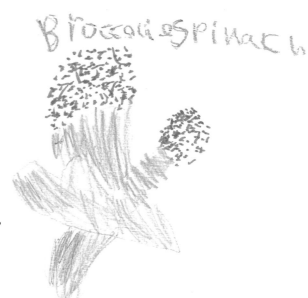

● The term 'boiling' is really a misnomer. Boiling often quickly becomes simmering, for if you boil something for any length of time, the pot would 'boil over'.

● If you boil protein, it hardens: you want that to happen to your breakfast boiled egg, but not to fish, meat or poultry. So stews or casseroles should be simmered – perhaps after bringing to the boil initially – on top of the stove or in the oven (solid-fuel cookers have specific simmering ovens).

● When boiling/simmering vegetables or meat, many of the nutrients leach into the water. Cook them in as little water as possible, and keep the water (it can be frozen in ice-cube trays and used as stock or to cook rice or other grains).

● Poaching is suitable for really delicate foods like fish and eggs, which cook through at a low temperature. When you poach eggs, add a little vinegar to the water before you add the eggs: this helps set the protein too. And if you poach fish in milk, say, keep the milk: it will be full of flavour, and can be used for an accompanying sauce (my poached smoked haddock in a cheese sauce, inside a pancake or pastry case, is a favourite; see page 162).

● Cook rice at a boil (or read the packet instructions), blanch green vegetables at a boil, and boil a liquid – stock, say – if you want to reduce its volume. Otherwise simmer or poach. You can simmer or poach in a low oven as well as on top of the stove (good for fruit). But why not cook vegetables you might normally boil in a completely different way: in a stir-fry (a little oil is used, but they will be full of texture and flavour), or in the oven (see page 57)?

Steaming

This is a better option than boiling, as it is gentler. Food is put in a double or triple pan, or a steaming basket in a saucepan. In effect, food is cooked in hot steam created by boiling water beneath it. Steaming takes a little longer than boiling as the food isn't in direct contact with heat, but nutrients are not lost in the water, and there is also less chance of overcooking a vegetable. I have a three-tier steamer, which I use all the time when I cook for the whole family. You can do a complete meal in a steamer: fish or chicken in the bottom, potatoes in the middle and vegetables on the top.

Frying and grilling

The main appeal of frying and grilling is that they create a 'burned' or 'caramelized' crust on the outside of the food, which adds flavour. Boiled, steamed or poached foods lack this, which is why they can sometimes be quite bland. Frying, especially deep-frying, is definitely the least healthy of all the cooking methods. However careful you are about coating a food (with breadcrumbs or batter) to protect it from fat and heat, or with draining it afterwards, fried food inevitably retains some of the fat it is cooked in. The smaller the item, the more fat it will contain and retain: the very thin fast-food French fries are *much* fattier than larger chips.

Grilling is a much healthier option, as there is no fat added, and indeed fat can drip out of a food such as a steak or chop during the cooking process. You can use an overhead or oven grill or you can buy a cast-iron ridged grill pan, which needs little fat, and gives foods attractive scorched stripes. But some nutritionists say that the caramelized outsides of fried or grilled foods can be carcinogenic. This is particularly true of barbecued foods, where the heat can be so much greater than that of a domestic grill.

I avoid deep-frying, but I do shallow-fry an egg occasionally. If shallow-frying, I try to use butter or olive oil (or a mixture), which I

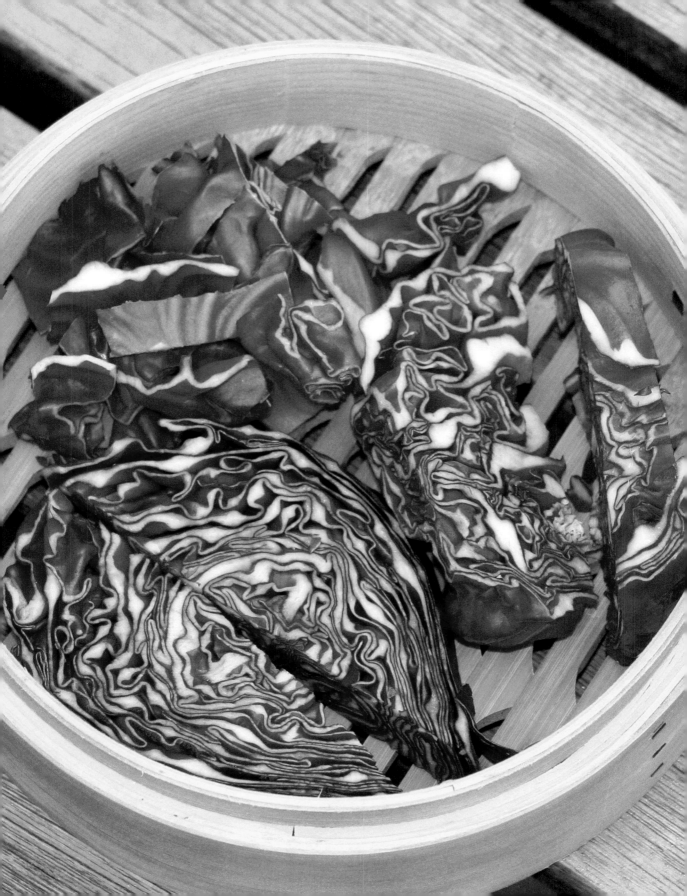

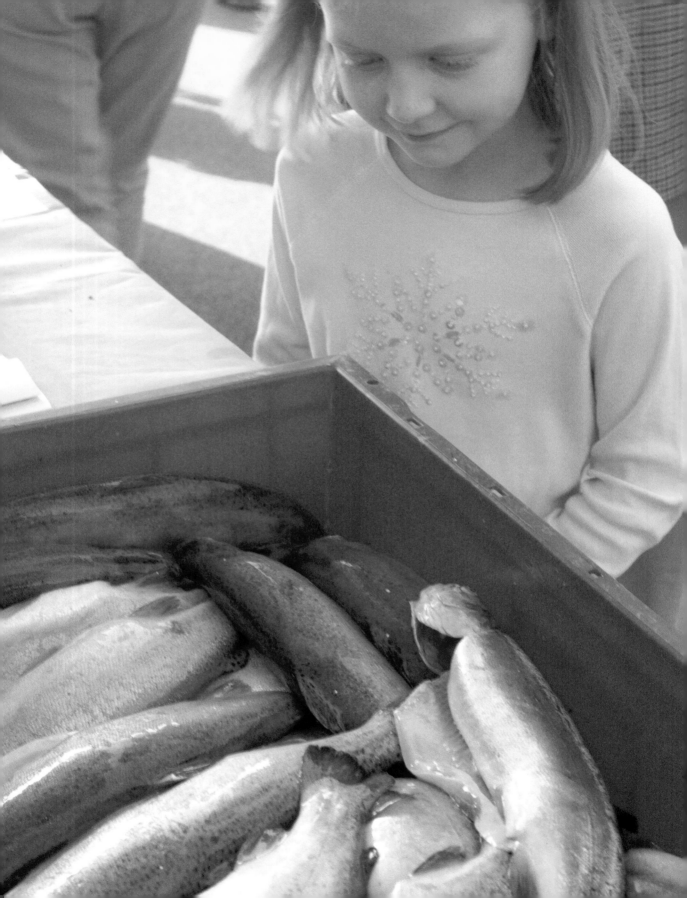

think is tastier than polyunsaturated vegetable oils. Stir-frying is much the same process, but you use very little oil: you cook the food at quite a high heat, uncovered, but for a very short time, so that it retains crispness. There is also a technique called steam-frying: you fry a food with a very small amount of oil and some liquid (water, stock or soy sauce) which, when the pan is covered, effectively steams the food. You can also buy special lidded pans, that are designed to steam foods in their own juices or 'fry' foods with no oil. And of course there are non-stick pans, which don't need any fat at all.

Baking/roasting

There is basically no difference between these terms these days: it means cooking in an enclosed oven at a fairly high heat (traditionally roasting was done on a spit in front of or over an open fire). Many things that you think you can only fry or grill can be cooked in the oven. The most traditional fish dish in Britain, for instance, is deep-fried battered fish. Sometimes I can hardly taste or appreciate the soft tasty flesh of the fish because of the crispness and oiliness of the batter. Roasting or baking plain fish in the oven at a high temperature is a much healthier, tastier and easier option. It takes no longer to cook, and all you really need to do is put a bit of butter, and possibly herbs, underneath or on top.

What would our Sunday lunch be without a roast potato?

Vegetables are good roasted plain or with other flavourings (see page 182), and what would our Sunday lunch be without a roast potato (I do try to use less fat these days)? A baked potato is one of my favourites – and it was on the menu at St Peter's every day. It is fat-free (unless you put lots of butter or cheese on top), and full of fibre and other nutrients. You can bake bacon in the oven until crisp (best on a rack so the fat drips away); and you can bake eggs in quite a few guises (see page 117–18), which is healthier than frying. Another baking trick – good with fish or vegetables – is to wrap food in lightly oiled foil (with other flavourings – herbs or lemon, for example), and bake. The foods bake and steam at the same time, losing none of their goodness or flavour.

Easier than you think

The following ideas are very simple indeed, but I hope they give you an idea of what can be done …

Sauce of infinite variety

Sauces are thought of as difficult, and as part of 'sophisticated' cooking, but there are two basic sauces that should be part of all good home cooking. I learned to make them when I did my cookery courses before the boys were born. They are both very easy – they're the same, just using a different base liquid – and once you have mastered the basic recipe you can adapt them in a variety of ways. Flour sauces aren't very fashionable these days in restaurant cooking, but are very handy when catering for children. Think of how many uses they have: coating cooked vegetables or hard-boiled eggs; in macaroni cheese and other pasta dishes; in the filling for pastry pies; as a topping for lasagne or moussaka; as a binding in croquettes; or as the basis of a soufflé. They can transform leftovers too, wonderful if you are in a hurry: combine vegetable and meat leftovers in an ovenproof dish, pour over a plain or flavoured sauce, sprinkle with cheese, and bake or grill until heated through.

Making a basic white sauce

As I'm sure you all know, a white sauce is a mixture of butter, plain flour and milk (you can use whole, semi-skimmed or skimmed milk). Melt the butter in a thick-bottomed pan, remove the pan from the heat, and stir in the flour until smooth and well combined. Return to the heat and cook for a minute. Do not let it brown. Remove from the heat again and add about a third of the milk, stirring continuously until smooth (warming the milk first helps to prevent lumps). Return the pan to the heat and stir, adding the rest of the milk gradually, and bring to the boil. Simmer for a couple of minutes, stirring, to allow the flour to cook through. That's it!

If you want to make the basic white sauce taste a little more interesting – in what is called a béchamel sauce – flavour the milk first. Put the milk in a small pan, add a few peppercorns, a slice of raw onion and a bay leaf (or anything you like), and bring nearly to the boil. Turn off the heat, and leave the milk and its flavourings to infuse for at least a couple of hours. Strain and use as in the basic recipe. The difference in flavour is amazing.

COOKING IN SCHOOLS

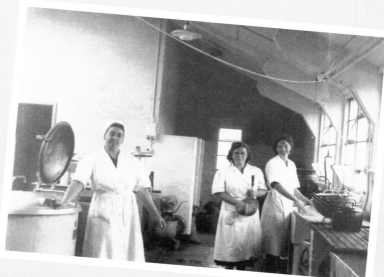

Old-fashioned domestic science and home economics – or hands-on cookery classes – are a thing of the past in most schools. Over the years cooking in schools became marginalized, until the early 1990s when food education began to be studied under the heading of 'Design and Technology'. Advocates of the new 'food technology' (oh, how I hate that term) say that the new syllabus injected fresh ideas into what had become a boring, if worthy, subject. I must admit that I didn't enjoy my cookery lessons at school, but then again, I wasn't as interested in food as I am now. As an example of food technology 'cooking', a friend of mine's daughter was studying food technology, and was going to be making a cheesecake. The 'recipe' was a packet of digestive biscuits (pre-crushed at home: there were no facilities at school), some butter and a box of that powdered whip stuff…

Even if I did not enjoy my classes, at least I got to handle some basic foodstuffs. One introduction to food technology states that students 'learn about hygiene and safety, nutrition, healthy eating and the correct use of tools and equipment. They are taught to prepare and try out their ideas in food product design lessons.' The latter sentence comes closest to 'cooking', but sadly it's much more likely to be how food technologists get new ideas. So our children learn little about real food, and as a result are totally disconnected from it. This was one of the most horrifying revelations of Jamie Oliver's TV programmes: the children who could not recognize basic fruit and vegetables.

If our children are to become healthy, well-fed adults, they must buy, cook and eat good food. If this is not learnt in the home, then must the schools bear the responsibility (yet another one)?

Cooking facilities are never a priority in cash-strapped schools, as they are expensive to install and maintain. But if the Government continues along its line of advocating better school dinners (improving school kitchens, training dinner ladies, allowing more money to be spent on ingredients), then some extra money should surely be allocated to teaching children about good food in a practical way.

Much has been done and achieved already. Many initiatives from chefs, food writers, supermarkets, charities and various other organizations have been trying to restore cookery lessons to the timetable. Some schools have re-introduced them, but this is by no means nationwide. They should be compulsory, as I believe that the earlier children are introduced to good food, the better – little chefs make better eaters. Some schools will have to spend money, but it will be worth it. In the long term, we could save the Government billions in NHS money now spent treating people with diet-related illnesses, and we could be helping the catering industry gain chefs of the future. But, most importantly, we would be raising children who are not entrenched in a fast-food culture, who are aware of the values and flavours of real food – and who, in turn, could teach their children the same lessons.

Making a velouté sauce

This is the French name for a sauce that is exactly the same as a white sauce, but which uses white stock (made from vegetables or uncooked bones, see page 223) instead of milk. This is the one that you would use with chopped-up vegetables and leftover chicken or meat as a pie filling.

You can make a darker sauce with a more intense flavour by using a brown stock. Make using a stock as described on page 223, but roast the meat or poultry bones and vegetables first. You can add a little tomato paste for extra colour.

Varying sauce thicknesses

Depending on the proportions, you can vary the thickness of a white, béchamel or velouté sauce, to use for different purposes.

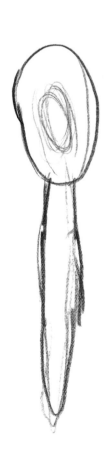

● A thin sauce, as the basis of a soup, say, uses 15g (¹/₂ oz) each of butter and flour to 300ml (10fl oz) milk or stock.

● A pouring sauce, for an accompanying sauce or gravy, uses 20g (³/₄ oz) butter and flour to 300ml (10fl oz) milk or stock.

● A coating sauce, for (obviously) coating and topping, uses 25g (1oz) butter and flour to 300ml (10fl oz) milk or stock.

● A binding sauce, for croquettes, soufflés etc., uses 55g (2oz) butter and flour to 300ml (10fl oz) milk or stock.

Flavouring sauces

At its simplest, you can add a pinch of freshly grated nutmeg to a white or béchamel sauce. But there are a number of ways in which any of these sauces can be flavoured.

● Onion (or shallot) sauce Gently cook 115g (4oz) sliced onions in a little more butter until soft, about 15 minutes, then continue as in the basic recipe. Good with poultry, lamb and vegetables.

● Mushroom sauce Gently cook 115g (4oz) mushrooms in a little more butter until soft, about 10 minutes, then continue as in the basic recipe for white or béchamel sauce. Good with fish, meat and poultry.

● **Cheese (or Mornay) sauce** Add 115g (4oz) grated Cheddar or other hard cheese to a white sauce off the heat at the end of cooking. Do not cook further. Good with chicken, eggs, fish, pasta (delicious with macaroni) and vegetables, and as the topping for lasagne and moussaka. You could use a blue cheese as well (but use less, 55g/2oz), which is good with steak, broccoli or pasta.

● **Herb sauce** Add 2–6 tablespoons chopped fresh herbs (parsley, tarragon, sage, etc) at the end of cooking. Good with bacon or gammon, fish, eggs and vegetables.

● **Mustard or horseradish sauce** Add 1–2 tablespoons mustard (French, Dijon or English, depending on the heat you like) or horseradish cream at the end of cooking. Good with vegetables to accompany a roast.

● **Egg sauce** Hard-boil 2 eggs, chop up and add to a white sauce at the end of cooking, along with a handful of chopped fresh parsley. Good with fish, and a great way of getting children to take in some extra protein.

● **Green sauce** Add about 115g (4oz) blanched chopped spinach or watercress to a white or béchamel sauce at the end of cooking.

● **Curried sauce** Add 1–2 tablespoons curry powder to the butter in the basic recipe, and a dash of lemon juice at the end. Good with hard-boiled eggs.

Mince it!

Mince is virtually the national dish of Scotland. My Scottish friend's mother used to serve mince with white pudding (an oat version of black pudding) on Saturdays, mince with 'tatties' (potatoes) on Tuesdays, and mince with curry power and raisins, with desiccated coconut sprinkled on top on Fridays (this was 'curry'). Mince can still be as varied, although I think we have more interesting ideas now. The suggestions below have got a distinct international flavour to them.

By 'mince' we usually mean beef, but of course any minced meat will do. Most supermarkets sell lamb and pork mince, and HRH the Prince of Wales is encouraging the wider availability of mutton which, minced, makes great shepherd's pie. Mince, certainly of beef, is generally made from the tougher cuts of meat such as silverside, blade, skirt, shin or neck. Although the process of mincing the meat breaks down the meat fibres and connective tissues, most mince still needs at least 35 minutes' cooking to tenderize it. So it's not necessarily a quick-fix meal, although if you buy better cuts from the butcher and asked him to mince them for you, it would cook rather more quickly.

Mince is a good source of protein (see page 80), and from experience I know that you can 'hide' vegetables in mince dishes and they're eaten by children who don't like them. At St Peter's, dishes made with mince were amongst the most popular: I think children like the texture as well as the taste, and there are no great lumps of meat to chew on, which can be quite daunting, especially for younger children. Mince can be rather high in fat, though really good-quality mince these days has very little fat in it. If you are concerned, dry-fry the mince in the pan by itself, drain the fat away and continue the recipe – adding the onions for example. Mince, because of its many surfaces, can potentially harbour bacteria if it has been hanging around. Buy it as freshly prepared as possible from a reliable butcher, use it as quickly as possible, and cook it thoroughly.

Most mince dishes are cooked as below, but meat loaves and meatballs are made with mince and then baked, grilled or fried. See page 128 for my hamburger loaf. Hamburgers are also made from raw minced meat, but from steak mince, which is better than ordinary butcher's mince.

Basic mince recipe

Mince needs a flavouring, and this can be onion alone, or onions and garlic, or onions, garlic, carrots and celery. I usually add to this half a green pepper and half a red pepper per 450g (1lb) mince, which will serve four people. Peel and chop the flavouring ingredients small, and fry gently until soft in a little vegetable or olive oil. Add the mince, and stir around in the pan, mixing it with the vegetables and oil, until the meat is brown (strain the fat off now if you want to). Then add liquid to cover – perhaps water with some Marmite or stock, or canned chopped tomatoes, depending on taste or the recipe – and any seasoning, flavourings or additions (if relevant). Cover and leave to simmer for 35–45 minutes, stirring occasionally. Season to taste. Boil up a little if too runny; add a little extra water or stock if too thick. Your basic mince is ready.

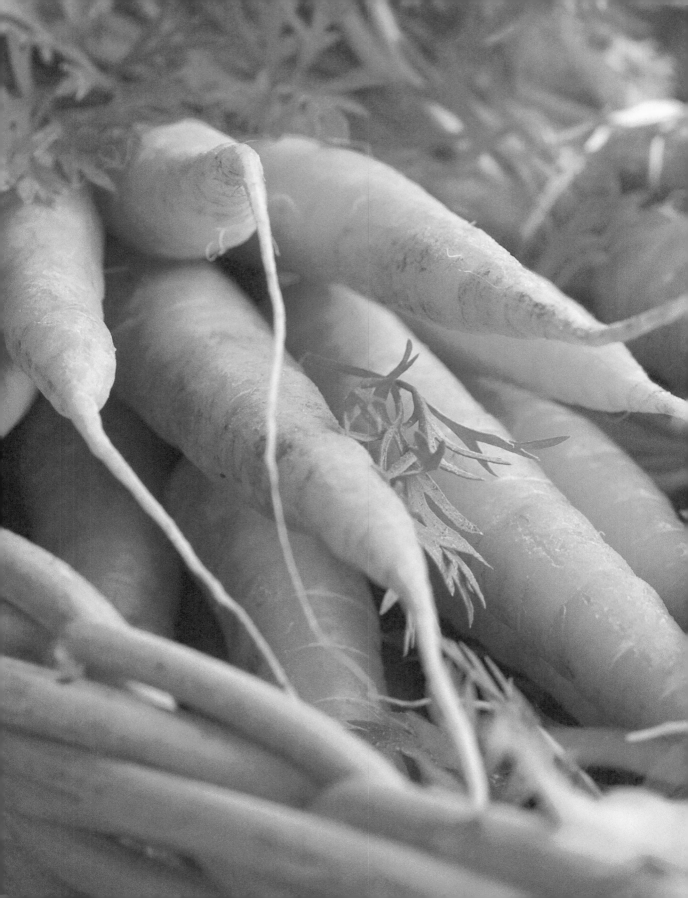

Varying your basic mince

Now you can try something different.

● **Cottage pie** Put the cooked (beef) mince in an ovenproof dish. Peel, cook and mash about 900g (2lb) potatoes, adding a little warm milk and butter (see page 194). Dot the top with more butter and bake in the preheated oven at 180°C/350°F/Gas 4 for about 25–30 minutes. (Or see my special cottage pie on page 137.)

● **Shepherd's pie** This is exactly the same, just made with lamb mince instead of beef.

● **Mince pie** Add other chopped vegetables to the mince – perhaps mushrooms, root vegetables, peas, sweetcorn, broccoli florets – along with a little more liquid if needed. Use to fill an ovenproof pie dish, and top with shortcrust (or puff) pastry. Bake in a preheated oven (about 220°C/425°F/Gas 7) for about 20 minutes or until the pastry is golden.

● **Chilli con carne** This is a spicy Mexican slant on mince (although the real recipe uses diced beef). Add a little chilli powder, ground cumin, dried oregano and tomato purée to the mince recipe while cooking. Add drained and rinsed canned red kidney beans, and heat through thoroughly. Serve with rice and/or tortilla chips – or wrap in a tortilla and serve with a spicy salsa.

● **Moussaka** This is Greek shepherd's pie, and is traditionally made with lamb. Layer your cooked mince with canned chopped or sliced fresh tomatoes, precooked sliced potatoes and shallow-fried or grilled slices of aubergine, coat with a cheese sauce (see page 61), and bake in a preheated oven at 200°C/400°F/Gas 6 for 25–30 minutes. You could mix the canned tomatoes in with the mince first. For a 'puffed' topping, add an egg yolk to the cheese sauce then fold in the whipped egg white before pouring on top of the mince and baking as above.

● **Lasagne** Layer the basic mince, which you will have cooked with tomatoes (add some dried herbs to it), with lasagne sheets (pre-cook if necessary, but the ready-to-use type is good), and a pouring cheese sauce (see page 61), finishing with sauce. Sprinkle with extra cheese. Bake at 200°C/400°F/Gas 6 for about 30 minutes.

● **Cannelloni** Stuff ready-to-use cannelloni tubes with a dryish cooked mince, arrange in a dish, and top with some pouring cheese sauce (see page 61). Bake as lasagne.

● **Bolognaise sauce** Our basic mince bears no real resemblance to an authentic Italian sauce, or ragù. They add pancetta or chicken livers, and cook the sauce for a very long time. However, the children at St Peter's loved my spaghetti bolognaise, which was the basic mince recipe with red and green peppers and mushrooms added, as well as a good pinch of dried mixed herbs.

● **Beef curry** Add some curry powder, or your own chosen mixture of fresh ground curry spices, at the beginning of cooking. Stir in some plain yoghurt and chopped fresh herbs at the end of cooking. Serve with rice and some raita (see page 234).

● **Stuffed vegetables** Instead of the rice mix on page 180, use some dryish mince to stuff tomatoes, peppers, aubergines, or courgettes. Bake as on page 180.

● **Stuffed leaves** Blanched Savoy cabbage (thick veins removed) or vine leaves can be wrapped around some dryish cooked mince, and then stewed gently in a tomato sauce until tender.

● **Mexican mince (enchilada)** Add some ground cumin and chilli powder to the basic mince and use it, fairly dry, as a stuffing for a tortilla. Serve with a spicy fresh salsa (see pages 230–32).

● **Mince pancakes** Buy or make large pancakes, stuff with the mince, and bake in a 200°C/400°F/Gas 6 oven, with a little grated cheese on top, for about 20 minutes.

● **Meat pasties** A dryish mince could be encased in a circle of pastry and sealed like a Cornish pasty. Bake in a preheated oven – 200°C/400°F/Gas 6 – for about 20 minutes until golden. You could do the same with those ready-to-bake vol-au-vent cases. Bake, then stuff with a hot, dryish mince.

HOME-MADE PASTRY

Making short-crust pastry for a pie topping or as a flan base is not nearly as difficult as you think.

225g (8oz) plain flour
55g (2oz) butter
55g (2oz) vegetable shortening
25ml (1fl oz) water

For wholemeal pastry use 175g (6oz) wholemeal flour and 55g (2oz) plain flour.

For sweet pastry add 25g (1oz) caster sugar.

● Put the flour in a large mixing bowl and rub the fats in until the mixture resembles fine breadcrumbs. Add the water and bring together with a knife until it forms a ball.

● Wrap in clingfilm, and put in the fridge to rest for about 30 minutes. Let the pastry come back to room temperature, then roll out thinly.

Blind baking

Sometimes you need to prepare flan cases before adding the filling. This is called blind baking.

● Preheat the oven to 200°C/400°F/Gas 6.

● Roll the pastry to fit your flan tin. Prick the base of the pastry case with the tines of a fork, then line with crushed greaseproof paper or foil, and fill with baking beans or dried pulses or rice (I keep some dried beans specially for blind baking).

● Place the tin in the oven for 10–15 minutes until the pastry looks set.

● Remove the paper or foil and beans, and bake for a further 5 minutes until the base is firm to the touch and lightly coloured. You don't want it to brown.

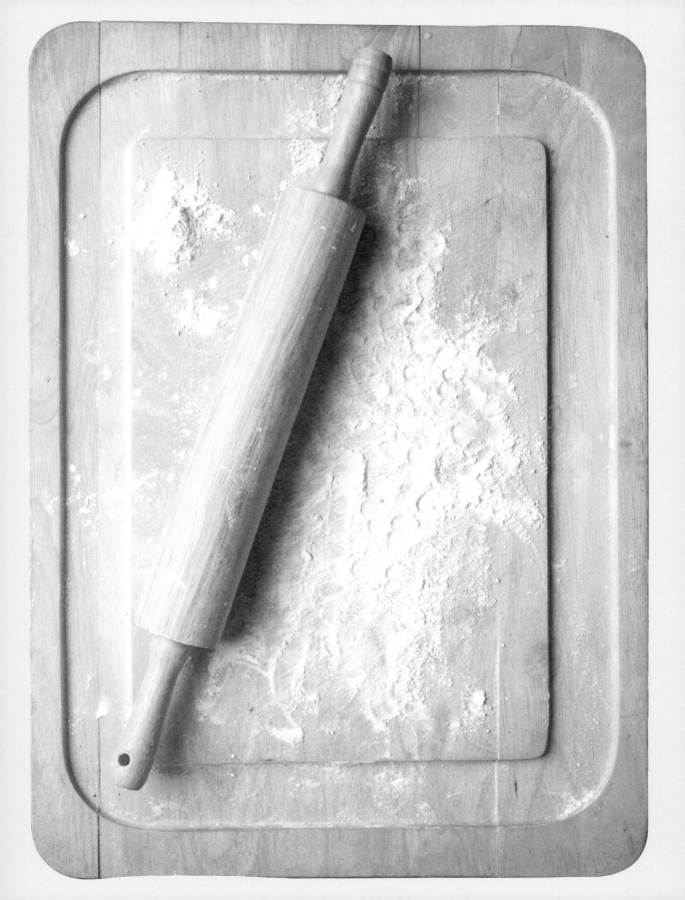

Cook now, eat later

If you are a busy parent you'll want to save and maximize your time, so that you have 'quality time' with your family. If you tend to come in exhausted from work, and want to have something quick to eat, don't resort to the ready meal and the microwave. If you are organized, you and your family can eat much more healthily. Firstly you need an hour or so dedicated to cooking (at the weekend probably), then your required tools are imagination (or a good recipe book such as this one, blowing my own trumpet!), your fridge and a good-sized freezer, perhaps a slow-cooker, and some airtight containers.

Cooking in advance and leftovers

We tend to forget one of the most basic facts, that many dishes can actually be prepared at least a day or two in advance. As long as your fridge is working properly, and you store things correctly – cold rather than warm, in a covered container – most foods will keep, whether raw or cooked (but not fish). In fact, some stews actually benefit from being left to 'mature' in the fridge: the flavour deepens, and you can lift any set fat off the surface. Reheat these dishes thoroughly.

Leftovers are perhaps the easiest aspect of the 'cook now, eat later' idea. If you have some leftover roast meat or poultry, then turn it into something else at a later time. Dorothy Hartley, in *Food in England*, tells of 'Vicarage Mutton', which was served 'hot on Sunday, cold on Monday, hashed on Tuesday, minced on Wednesday, curried on Thursday, broth on Friday, cottage pie on Saturday'. That must have been quite some joint to start with, but the basic concept is correct. It just does make sense to buy a bigger piece of meat than will serve one meal only. It saves time and money.

Cold meat and salad might be the easiest option, but you can mince the meat leftovers to make croquettes or rissoles; you could use beef or lamb in a cottage or shepherd's pie (see page 137); or make a pie with poultry or meat, minced or diced, vegetables and cheese sauce (see page 61) and a pastry topping; or stuff vegetables (see page 180) with leftovers. Make a stock with meat bones and poultry carcasses (see page 223), and freeze it, or use as the basis for a soup (see page 224). Leftover fish, such as salmon, can be quickly made into fishcakes (see page 167), which can be frozen too. Leftover vegetables, such as cabbage and potatoes (even Brussels sprouts), can be mashed or chopped together and fried or baked as bubble and squeak (see page 196).

Even leftover stale bread can be utilized. Either blend to crumbs and freeze (great for coating fishcakes or fish fillets, for stuffing, making rissoles, or a bread sauce), or slice it and make it into a bread or bread and butter pudding (add raisins, sugar, milk and flavourings).

Batch cooking

If you are going to spend time baking a cake, why not spend a little longer making more than one? The same applies to biscuits and breads. To make up enough mixture for two or more cakes or bread loaves takes no extra time, although the baking probably will take a little longer, depending on your oven. But you will have one to eat now, and a second or more to eat later (great if your kids are in the habit of bringing friends home for tea). Cool as quickly as possible, and then store one in an airtight box for a week or so, or freeze, un-iced, wrapped tightly in foil and freezer-wrap. Tray-bake cakes – mixtures baked in a baking tray – are good cut into small pieces and frozen. Because the pieces are small, they also defrost very fast. You can make two or three times the quantity of the cheese twist biscuits on page 244, for instance, and store some in an airtight box, layers separated with foil, or freeze them. They will need refreshing in a warm oven before serving to crisp them up, whether stored in box or freezer.

A large amount of tomato sauce takes little more time to cook than a smaller amount, and casseroles, soups and stocks are the same. When you are making a casserole, for instance, make a really big one, enough for double the number you usually cater for. Freeze half of it in a suitable dish, and you will have it there for the following week. You can even decant it from the dish once it is frozen and return it to the freezer in a bag, freeing the dish for another use. With sauces, soups, and stock, store what you don't need immediately, when cooked and cooled, in as many 300ml (10fl oz) yoghurt pots or freezer containers as you require, and freeze. You can also batch-cook and freeze baby food (see below).

There is so much that you can make in larger quantities and keep or freeze, so maybe one week in two you won't have to cook when you come home, but at least you know what you are eating.

Freezing

A freezer is magic for those of us who are busy. You can batch-cook (see above) one weekend afternoon or weekday evening, and freeze dishes in handy portions. George relies on the freezer during the week when I am away, taking out dishes one of us prepared earlier.

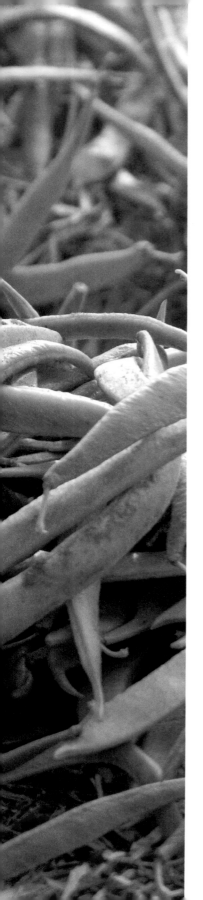

I talked about freezing in my last book, so I won't go into too much detail here. But use the freezer as an extra store-cupboard, and you will save loads of time – as long as you remember to take whatever you want well in advance! I buy bread and butter, for instance, in the local shops, and freeze them. If I'm cooking for a big occasion, like Christmas, say, I'll make and freeze several items in advance – mince pies, and turkey stuffing, for example.

When the boys were babies, I used to make up batches of salt- and sugar-free fruit and vegetable purées and freeze them in ice-cube trays. Then, when I wanted an apple purée for a hungry baby, I would take out one cube and heat it up. Good for the baby, and no waste!

You can freeze a glut of home-grown runner beans to enjoy later when they are out of season: blanch them first to help retain their colour, flavour and texture. Fresh fruit like raspberries freeze well too: open-freeze on a tray, then put them into freezer bags in handy portion sizes. Fruit sauces (see page 268) freeze very well (especially popular with the children as ice-lollies), even a strawberry sauce (whole fresh strawberries have too high a water content to freeze successfully).

Slow-cooking

This is stretching the 'cook now, eat later' idea, but I couldn't do without my slow-cooker – or 'crockpot' as it is sometimes called. It produces what is the complete opposite of 'fast food'! It's a large casserole that sits inside an electric base, which is used to cook soups and stews with a slow, moist heat. Slow-cookers are very useful – and make the best stock possible, with the liquid just at a murmur for hours, extracting every drop of flavour from the stock ingredients. The idea is to fry the meat and vegetables first, and add liquid, then leave it, covered, for 4–6 hours (that is 'fast') or for up to 12 hours ('slow'). You could even put it on the night before, leave it through the whole day, and when you come home at night you have a meal ready and waiting – and, of course, a lovely smell as you walk through the door!

Slow-cookers are very economical to run, as they only use the same amount of power as a light bulb, but they save you in other ways too. You can buy the cheaper cuts of meat such as brisket, shin, oxtail or mutton that benefit from a long, slow cooking time.

Do you really need to cook?

No, of course you don't. There are plenty of foods and dishes you can buy that are pre-cooked (and I *don't* mean ready meals), or that don't *need* to be cooked. The healthiest diet, in fact, according to many nutritionists, is one that has a large proportion of raw or very lightly cooked food; we should really have something raw with every meal for the best balance (see pages 79–83 for more advice on diet).

Raw foods retain most of their nutrients (depending on their age, of course), and they are full of texture, which most of us like, particularly children. Joanna Blythman, in *The Food Our Children Eat*, suggests that offering crunchy raw vegetables to reluctant vegetable-eaters is 'the most certain way to break down a vegetable veto'. Now that's something to think about!

Raw foods

Fruit is the first thing that springs to mind, and most are best eaten raw. I always kept a bowl of fresh fruit on the table when the boys were young, so they could help themselves to an apple, pear, plum, orange, tangerine or a bunch of grapes if they were hungry. A plate of fresh fruit cut into small pieces is the best snack when children come home from school. In the summer, you have a huge choice – strawberries and raspberries, as well as imported peaches and nectarines. Gooseberries and currants are good too, but they might need to be cooked, as they are quite tart: simmer briefly with a minimum of sugar. You could make a summer pudding with some of those berries, which is one of my favourite puddings (see page 264).

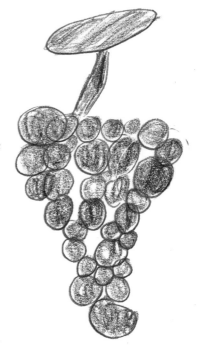

I like to try more exotic fruit too. Kiwis are almost too common to be called exotic any more, and they are packed full of vitamin C. They can be peeled and sliced into savoury or fruit salads, or they can be eaten ripe like a boiled egg, hat off, with a spoon, which amuses younger children. Pawpaws or papayas with seeds removed and a dash of lime juice make a good breakfast, as do mangoes, stone removed, the thick slices cross-hatched and turned over to make a 'hedgehog'. If you serve fruit as a pudding – in the hand, as a fruit salad, or with yoghurt or ice-cream – as a matter of course from the very earliest stages, no-one will hanker after anything stodgier and sweeter.

Vegetables are good raw too. Chunks of raw vegetables can be used as crudités to dip into a home-made or bought dip, salsa or guacamole (see pages 229–35). Children like to eat things with their fingers. They'll also eat raw cabbage in coleslaw much more readily than they would steamed cabbage with roast meat. I think it must be the texture. There are few vegetables that can't be eaten raw: carrots, cauliflower, peppers and tomatoes are obvious, but leeks and Brussels sprouts, for instance, if shredded finely enough, can be eaten raw in a salad.

And it is of course salads that are what most of us think of as 'raw food'. You could serve a salad every day of the week if you had the necessary ingredients, and each one could be different; there are so many possible combinations. Salad leaves are usually the basis, but avoid those packets of leaves, or 'gas-bags' as I call them (they've been washed in chlorine, puffed up with 'modified air', and are outrageously expensive). Buy a good lettuce, and a bunch of watercress or rocket, remove any tired outside leaves and wash the remainder. Spin in a salad spinner (a good investment if you eat a lot of salad), or dry on clean tea-towels or kitchen paper. Then start assembling. Use carrots, celery (even peeled celeriac diced very small), avocado, tomato, cucumber, peppers, broccoli, cauliflower – the list is endless. Vary the textures by grating, dicing, shaving or cutting into strips. Don't forget about fruit in savoury salads either: sliced orange, apple or peach adds flavour, colour, texture and sweetness. Dried fruit is useful too – mangoes, apricots, dates, raisins, sultanas – as are nuts and seeds (you could dry-fry these first to give them a toasted flavour).

Other no-cook ingredients

However, this is not just about fruit and vegetables. No-cook foods include other things that you can buy ready-prepared, that taste good, save you time, and, in combination with the raw foods mentioned above, make a good dish or meal. I'm thinking about cans of fish or shellfish and pulses, cheeses, cooked or cured ham etc. (In August 2005 it was reported that the Government is to conduct new research into the level of mercury in fish, amid claims that children who eat too much tuna may develop learning difficulties. You have to ask yourself, what is safe to eat?) A couple of slices of Parma ham with some melon or a sliced ripe pear is delicious. Sticks of celery stuffed with plain or flavoured cream cheese are full of flavour and crunch – a great after-school snack.

We've talked about salads, but you could add ready-prepared protein as well, to make a main course. Mix drained canned tuna or crab into a mixed salad, or chunks of cheese (children like Cheddar or mozzarella cheeses, even feta). Ribbons of ham or other leftover meat are good too. Canned pulses, such as kidney beans and chickpeas, are excellent, as they save so much time: rinse them well, drain, and add to a vegetable salad for additional protein and carbohydrate.

New flavours

One of the objects of this book is to try to help you broaden your children's palates, and so you could add other little touches for flavour, texture and colour. These could be anchovies, capers, fresh herbs or olives. I've always found the art of getting children to try new things is never to make a fuss. Buy a very small amount of any or all of the above, and instead of mixing them into a dish from the start, which might cause trouble, put in small bowls on the table beside the salad or whatever, and let the children help themselves if they want to.

With imagination, sensible planning and buying, and a fairly well-stocked store-cupboard, you can feed your family well without having to cook at all! It will also be much healthier – and cheaper – than some meat in an instant cooking sauce, a chilled ready meal, or a fast-food takeaway.

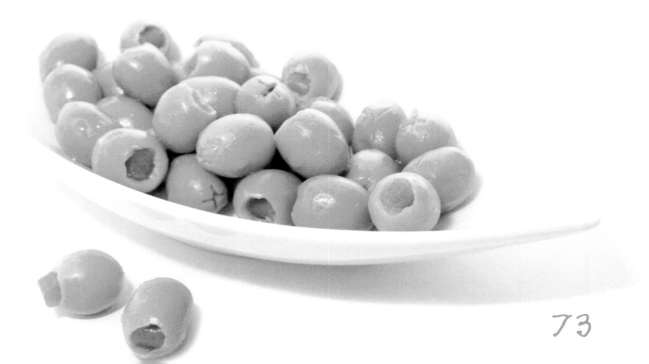

DINNER LADIES AND COOKING

I am very excited about my latest project. Since the middle of 2004 I have been working with Jim Collins, farmer, and Gary Stokes, farm manager, at Ashlyns Organic Farm in Essex. The farm comprises about 1,800 acres, and sells organic produce in three farm shops. In addition they have an educational centre open to the public, they organize school visits (so children learn about organic farming, and meet the animals), and they have set up a growing co-operative (with other local farmers growing and supplying vegetables to schools in the area).

Over the last 18 months or so we have planned, devised, designed and set up a cookery school especially for dinner ladies. We gave our first lessons in July 2005, and the school was formally opened in October by Jamie Oliver.

Gary was supplying about ten local schools with organic produce when I first met him in 2003. I gave a talk at Ashlyns, and then they asked me to become involved with them. We found that the school caterers and catering managers who were buying Ashlyns' products needed some guidance because they were not used to coping with fresh food. So we applied to the Department of Environment Food and Rural Affairs (Defra) for money to help us explore the idea of a training centre for school catering people. After months of negotiation, Defra agreed, and the plans began to take shape. I designed a working demonstration kitchen, but it's not an all-singing, all-dancing electronic affair. It's similar to a school kitchen, with very basic equipment. We employed a full-time development and training chef, Simon Owen, who worked on *Jamie's Dinners*, helping the schools in Greenwich. He and I work together to try and show the catering staff that this is not only about the food on the plate, it is the ethos of the Food for Life campaign, which I have always maintained has to be a whole-school approach. I believe catering staff cannot be responsible if they have no input into the food they are serving. So local authorities, the people they employ within the kitchens, head teachers, governors, parents and, most importantly, the children themselves should come together to make food part of education.

The training kitchen has huge potential. We have even been approached to run a course for young adults leaving care. We hope to show them how to shop and cook, which will give them an introduction to good nutritious food and eating. We aim to utilize the conference centre, and invite school governors, head teachers and teachers, who all need to know about the benefits of training their cooks and of fresh and organic food. The children won't be forgotten, as they can still visit the education centre and the farm, have lunch and enjoy their day out. For some it will be their first taste of fresh or organic food. The only person who misses out is my husband George, for I am rarely at home . . .

From top left, clockwise: **Being interviewed for local television; with Jamie Oliver and Simon Owen; Steve getting the mash ready; Jamie looking at some fresh produce; Jamie officially opening the kitchen with the local schoolchildren; and Kerry preparing lunch.**

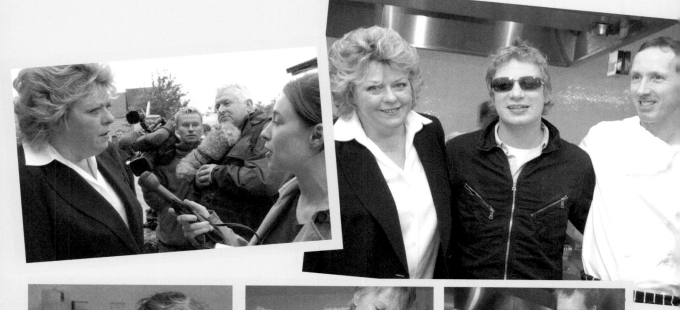
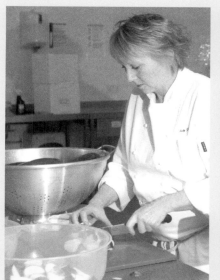
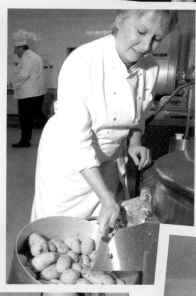
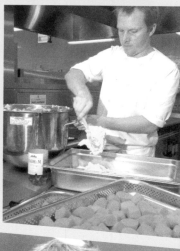
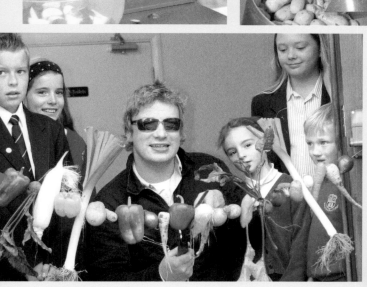
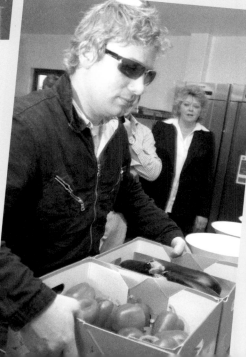

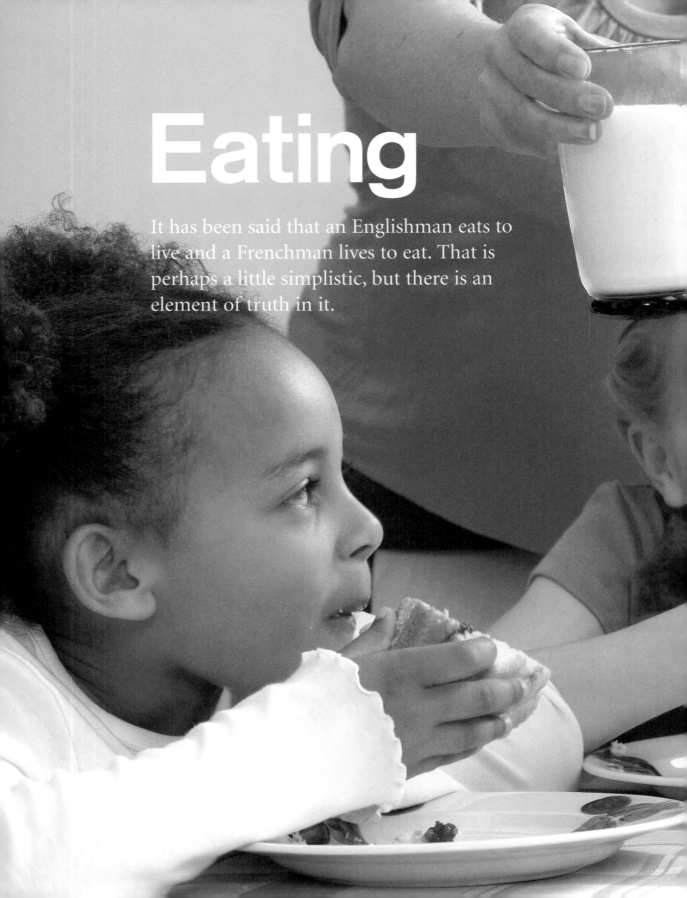

Eating

It has been said that an Englishman eats to live and a Frenchman lives to eat. That is perhaps a little simplistic, but there is an element of truth in it.

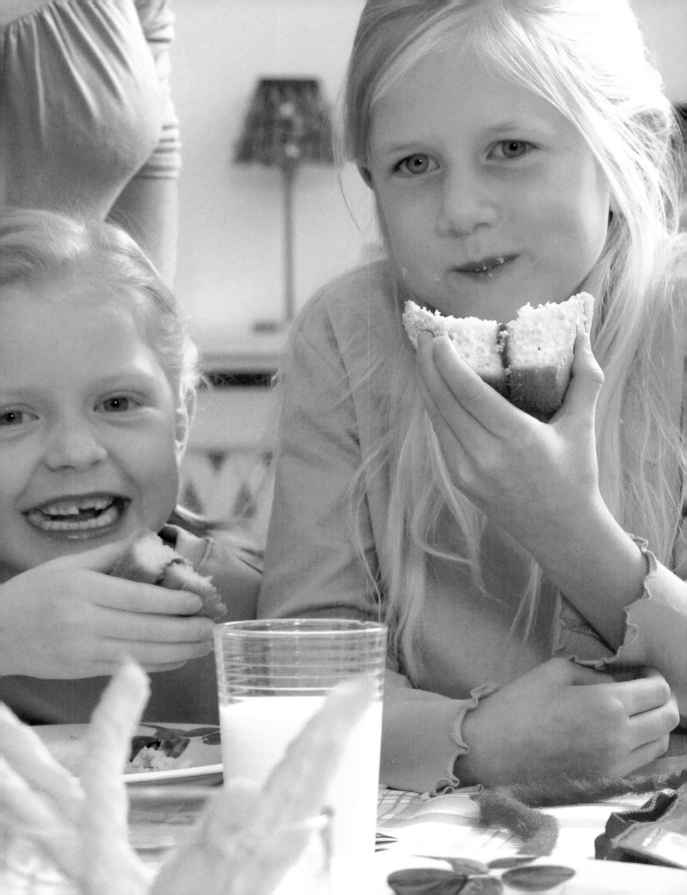

ALTHOUGH MANY of us love food in the UK, the general perception on the Continent – with our ready meals, lack of spending on school dinners, our snack and fast-food culture – is that we don't. I wish we were more like the French and Italians, with a centuries-old appreciation of good food and good eating together. But we seem to have gone in another direction. The trend is beginning to reverse, but it is a slow process.

Eating is one of life's pleasures. A beautifully cooked meal in pleasant surroundings, with the family around you, is something to treasure. When the children grow up and move away it all changes, and it seems very strange to me now to be cooking only for two or three instead of five or six. My husband says I still cook too much, but old habits die hard. I miss sitting around a table discussing the day's events with the boys, even the arguments. I must admit I'm looking forward to my grandchild, Jacob James, coming to stay, and I am so looking forward to his first Christmas. In my mind I have it planned already – although he will only be four months old. Oh well, there'll be plenty of time to teach him to cook and eat properly, I hope.

The pleasure of eating is all about flavour or taste. Children have very acute taste-buds, more so than adults, because the number of taste-buds declines with age. Flavour is in fact a combination of taste, smell, texture and other physical features such as temperature. At least 50 per cent of what is perceived as taste is smell. To test this, hold your nose, close your eyes, and try to taste the difference between coffee and tea, red wine and white wine, or grated apple and onion. I guarantee you won't be able to. Your children might enjoy this too, but choose the test tastes carefully!

Why food is important

These days it is vitally important to think about what we give our children to eat. The food industry offers plenty of fast foods, ready meals, even foods specially designed for children, but there is evidence that many of these are contributing to our children's ill health and obesity. Fresh food is the answer, but your cooking of it has to compete with the blandishments of cartoon-inspired, highly sugared cereals, hamburgers and fries, processed cheesy dips, and desserts.

You have to work hard to sway children in your own healthy direction (starting early is one strategy, see below), but if you can involve them in healthy buying and cooking, you should be able to involve them in healthy eating as well.

The building blocks of food

Fresh foods contain the most nutrients, and children – as well as adults – need to balance the combination of these nutrients on a daily basis. The Balance of Good Health should be your guide (see page 82). The basic building blocks of food are carbohydrates, proteins and fats. Most of the foods that contain them will also provide essential vitamins and minerals.

Carbohydrates

These provide energy and keep you warm. Carbohydrates are found primarily in cereals, starchy foods (such as potato) and grains (such as rice). They are grouped into two categories, simple and complex. This division indicates the speed at which they are broken down into blood sugar or glucose (the main fuel of the body). Complex carbohydrates are the best, as they break down slowly, therefore producing energy for longer. Simple carbohydrates or sugar are broken down and used very rapidly in the body. A good breakfast of porridge or wholegrain cereal (complex carbohydrate) keeps your child going for longer than a bowl of highly sweetened, processed cereal.

Good sources of complex carbohydrate include potatoes, wholemeal bread and pasta, brown and white rice, and whole unsweetened cereals. Many of these carbohydrate foods also contain fibre, which keeps your digestive system working.

Proteins

Meat, fish, poultry, eggs, dairy foods, pulses, nuts and Quorn are good sources of protein. Proteins, often known as the bricks and mortar of the body, are required for the development of almost everything, including the brain and nervous system. Protein is important for children for growth. Protein is made up of amino acids and animal protein is the most 'complete'; vegetable proteins are not 'complete', so need to be eaten in combination (grains and beans, for example). Eating vegetable proteins in conjunction with animal protein can work well nutritionally – bread and cheese, cereal with milk, spaghetti with a bolognaise sauce. Many foods which are rich in protein contain other nutrients – red meats and oily fish, for instance, contain iron, which children especially need.

The best proteins for children are dairy foods (milk, cheese, eggs, natural bio-live yoghurt), meat, poultry, fish, pulses (especially soya beans and products made from them, such as tofu) and grains. Nuts are a good source of protein, but take care because some children are allergic to them. Nuts should never be offered to very young children, both because of the allergy possibility, and also because they might choke.

Fats

We all need fats, especially children at times of major growth. They are important for brain and nerve development, amongst other things, which is why children under two years old should have whole milk. Some vitamins are fat-soluble, so can't be absorbed without fat. However, we need the right type, and everyone is encouraged to eat more unsaturated fats, particularly monounsaturated fats such as rapeseed or olive oil. Certain polyunsaturated fats are further divided into Omega-6 and Omega-3 essential fatty acids. Omega-6-rich foods include avocado, corn, seeds (particularly sesame and sunflower), nuts and grains. Omega-3-rich foods include some seeds (pumpkin), wheat, beans, nuts and spinach, as well as fish (especially oily fish such as fresh salmon, tuna, sardines and mackerel).

Saturated fats, the ones we should be careful about, are found in animal products such as meat, fish and dairy wholefoods, but also in palm oil (used in the food industry). Saturated fats can contribute to raised cholesterol levels in the blood vessels, which can lead to heart disease. Some healthy fats become saturated fats through processing – trans fats and hydrogenated fats – and these are widely used in the food industry as well. These fats not only contribute to ill-health and obesity,

WILLOWS
SEAFOOD

Y

D SEAFOOD

			SEA BASS	lbs
			SEA BREAM	£5-7
			MULLET (RED)	
			MULLET (GREY)	
lbs	kgs.		PLAICE	
ARKED	600		(DOVER)	AS MARKED

THE BALANCE OF GOOD HEALTH

The Balance of Good Health is a pictorial food guide produced by the Food Standards Agency to help us understand how to eat healthily. Shaped like a dinner plate, the guide is divided into five sections which show, in a clear visual way, the proportion and types of foods that are needed to make up a healthy balanced diet. There is no complicated measuring of portions, which can be confusing, and the guide shows that you do not have to give up any food you enjoy: all foods can be part of a healthy diet, so long as they are in overall balance.

The five food groups are: 1) fruit and vegetables; 2) bread, other cereals and potatoes; 3) milk and dairy foods; 4) meat, fish and alternatives such as poultry, offal, nuts, eggs, vegetable proteins and beans; 5) foods containing fat and foods containing sugar. Sections 1 and 2 are the largest, therefore these foods should form a major part of the daily diet. Sections 3 and 4 are smaller, so moderate amounts of these foods should be eaten daily. Section 5 is the smallest, so foods from this group should be eaten in very small amounts daily.

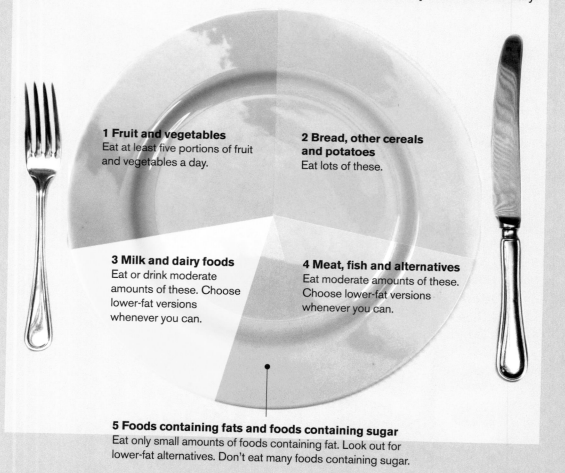

1 Fruit and vegetables
Eat at least five portions of fruit and vegetables a day.

2 Bread, other cereals and potatoes
Eat lots of these.

3 Milk and dairy foods
Eat or drink moderate amounts of these. Choose lower-fat versions whenever you can.

4 Meat, fish and alternatives
Eat moderate amounts of these. Choose lower-fat versions whenever you can.

5 Foods containing fats and foods containing sugar
Eat only small amounts of foods containing fat. Look out for lower-fat alternatives. Don't eat many foods containing sugar.

NB The Balance of Good Health does not apply to children under the age of five years.

82

but also hinder absorption of the healthy fats. Foods that are high in hydrogenated fats include shop-bought cakes, biscuits, margarines, some pizzas, turkey twizzlers, and chicken nuggets. (Another reason to make your own nuggets.) Don't offer children low-fat or 'lite' versions of foods, though, as these are highly processed.

Vitamins and minerals

These are very important nutrients found in different amounts in a variety of foods, especially fresh foods. They are essential to children's growth and development and the health of adults. By eating a wide variety of different foods you will get all the vitamins and minerals you need. Some vitamins can deteriorate as soon as food is harvested (which is why fresh local food that has not travelled too far, or freshly frozen food, is a better source of some vitamins such as Vitamin C). Some vitamins are destroyed by heat or exposure to air, and it is important not to chop and prepare ingredients a long time before cooking them. Each one has a particular job to do: Vitamin A (in eggs, dairy foods and especially orange vegetables and fruit) helps eyes, skin and teeth; the Vitamin B group (in whole grains, fish, pulses, eggs and nuts) turns food into energy, good for the nerves, muscles, skin, and digestive system; Vitamin C (in citrus fruits, vegetables, and other fruit) helps the body absorb iron, and heals wounds; Vitamin D (in fish and eggs) helps your body absorb calcium, and is good for bone development; Vitamin E (in whole grains, leafy green vegetables, eggs and some fish) helps the body make blood cells and looks after body tissues.

The really key minerals are: iron (in red meat, oily fish such as sardines, eggs, pulses and green leafy vegetables), which is essential to the making of red blood cells, and calcium (in dairy foods, canned salmon and sardines – with bones – and dried fruit), which is essential for teeth and bone development. Children need a lot of calcium when going through their growth spurts. Salt is also a mineral, and it is important that you don't eat too much (6g a day for adults, 2g for one-to-two-year-olds, 3g for four-to-six-year-olds, 5g for seven-to-ten olds). Some processed foods contain a lot of salt – particularly ready-prepared sauces and soups, some ready-made dishes, salted snacks, smoked foods and some canned foods.

Fat or fit?

We are told that the child obesity statistics are horrifying – one in ten six-year-olds is obese, and the number of dangerously overweight children has doubled since the early 1980s. A fat child will probably become a fat adult, and thus increase the risks of early heart disease, stroke and diabetes. Children in their teens are now falling victim to type-2 diabetes, previously a disease of adults. The established view is that this is due to the 'immobility' of our TV generation of children, but obesity is a result of both inactivity and eating more energy than is used up each day. Children these days spend more time sitting in front of a TV or computer screen, and may eat more foods such as crisps, snacks and ready meals which can contribute to greater energy intake.

● If you are overweight, your child is 80 per cent more likely to become overweight too. Why? Because there are usually more fatty foods and sugary snacks in the house. Set your children a good example by not eating junk foods yourself, and buying lots of fruits and vegetables for snacking.

● Many parents find it difficult to get their child to eat anything; others have children who eat whatever comes their way. The majority of children know when they have had enough, and leave food on their plates, but some carry on eating until their plate is empty even after they are full. If you are concerned about how much your child eats, make sure their meals follow the BGH guidance (see page 82).

● Give kids a good breakfast (see page 104). This starts the day off well, and will prevent them having the 'munchies' halfway through the morning, when they would probably choose something sugary to replenish flagging energy. Apart from being bad for them, this might spoil their appetite for lunch; if they don't eat enough lunch, they may seek out more sugary foods during the afternoon, spoiling their appetite for a healthy tea or supper. It's a vicious circle.

● Children are growing, so should never be put on a diet: even the most severely obese children are given a restrictive diet only under close medical supervision. Worrying about fat and calories can lead young minds to guilt, unhappiness, lack of self-esteem and obsession, and perhaps to the diet diseases anorexia and bulimia (which can affect both girls and boys). Rather than restricting quantity, which could lead to a lack of nutrients necessary for growing bodies, focus on healthy foods and limit foods that lack quality.

● Eating together as a family – one of my passions – is one way of ensuring kids (and adults) avoid obesity. If you all eat healthy food together, the temptation for children to snack at other times is reduced. If one member of the family is overweight, eating the same food as everyone else prevents them feeling 'singled out' (which they might be if you prepared and cooked separate dishes for them).

● Take more exercise as a family. We seem to be demonizing our children, saying they do not take enough exercise. To encourage your children, be active yourself. Play rugby, football, cricket or go swimming with them – or, if you're not too sports minded, simply go for a walk. A family walk before Sunday lunch will work off a few calories, exercise joints, and build up a collective appetite. Walk the children to school. See www.walktoschool.org.uk, which has some interesting ideas (about health, fitness, bone density, sociability and reducing driving and school traffic jams).

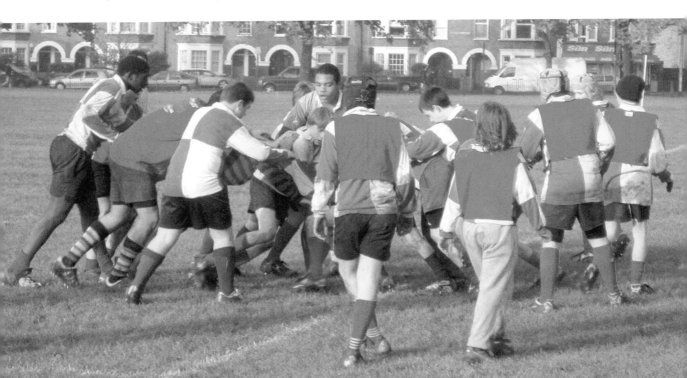

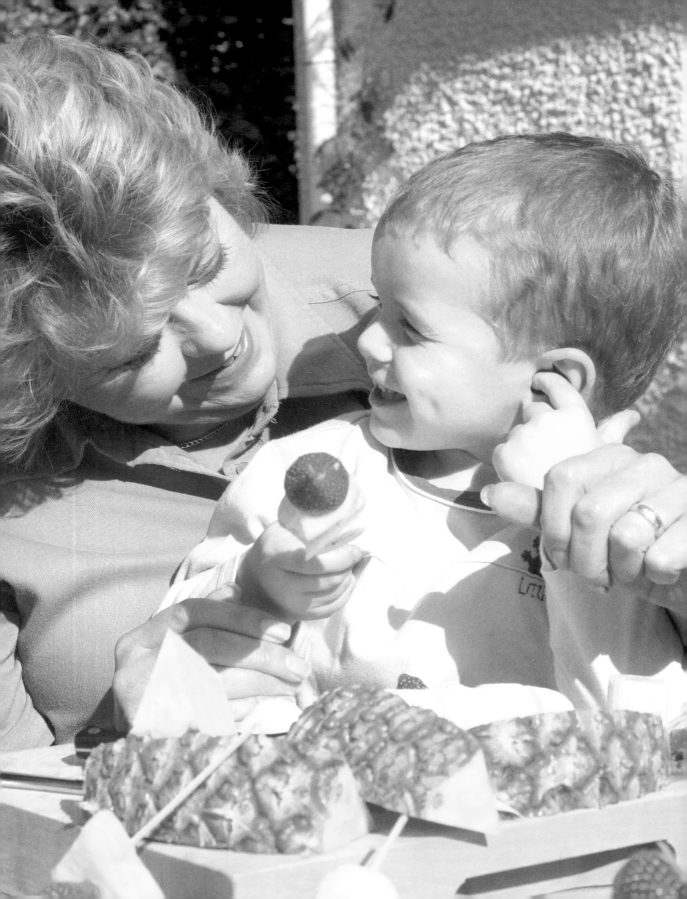

When eating well is most important

Eating good food is important throughout all our lives, but it is particularly so for children, especially during the major periods of growth: in the womb; during the first couple of years; and during puberty and adolescence.

During pregnancy

Eating well during pregnancy means that you give your baby the best possible start in life. You only have nine months in which to do it, so virtually every mouthful will count. You are literally 'eating for two', but that doesn't mean enough for two adults. An average woman needs about 1940 kcals a day, and she does not need to eat more until the last trimester, when a small (200 kcals) extra a day are recommended. Never put yourself on any sort of diet, thinking you might become overweight after pregnancy; if you limit what you eat, you limit the food your baby eats.

Those calories you eat should be of the best quality possible, from fresh, preferably organic foods from all the major building blocks (see pages 79–83). Concentrate on vitamin- and mineral-rich foods, because your baby needs nutrients like calcium (drink milk, eat almonds, dried apricots, etc.), iron (eat dried fruit, beef, sardines), and Vitamin C (eat citrus fruit or yellow or green fruits and vegetables). Drink plenty of water, as your baby's body, like yours, is composed of water (see page 100). Avoid alcohol, drinks such as tea and coffee, which contain caffeine, and cut down on salt and sugar.

During early childhood

On average, babies double their birth weight by the age of six months, and triple it by their first birthday. That is a lot of growth in a very short space of time. Breast milk is best for babies, as it contains all the essential nutrients and passes on antibodies to the child. A breast-feeding mother should eat a good diet – around an extra 500 kcals a day to produce milk – and drink plenty of water, as this will ensure her own health and milk flow are at their best (for this is rather an exhausting time!).

By six months an infant's nutritional needs cannot be met by milk alone, and you should start to wean – with rice cereal first (because of possible allergies), then small tastes of vegetable and fruit purées, soft

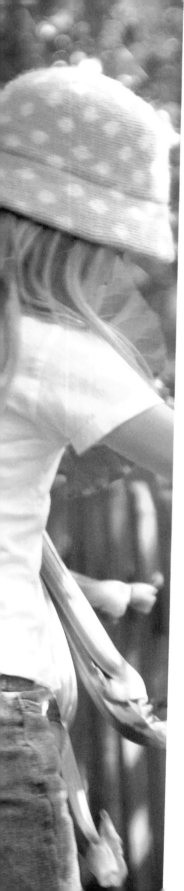

meat, fish and pulses, unsalted and unsweetened. Try to vary tastes as the baby gets older.

By the age of one year, your baby's diet should consist mostly of solid foods, although milk still has a place. Energy requirements will have risen because of the child's quick growth at this stage – and his or her increasing level of activity once crawling and then walking start. At this age children should be having three small meals a day as well as milk drinks. After one, children will need snacks between meals as well. Make these snacks healthy – pieces of fruit or cheese, dried fruit, yoghurt – and you will establish a healthy eating pattern for life. Calorie requirements sometimes drop at some stage in the child's second year as growth is slowest between 15–18 months and four years. Good food is obviously important, but don't overfeed: trying to 'feed up' young children can actually make them grow out rather than up, causing them to become chubbier, not taller.

Trying to 'feed up' young children can actually make them grow out rather than up.

During adolescence

The second major growth spurt occurs during adolescence. Girls start this earlier, usually between seven and ten, and boys later, between ten and 14. Teenage boys can grow as much as 9cm (3½ inches) a year, and teenage girls 8cm (3in) a year. This, however, is also the time when children are most influenced by TV advertising and by peer pressure. Protein is important for growth, as are fresh fruit and vegetables. The rapid increase in bone mass at this stage means calcium-rich foods are particularly valuable (cheese, milk, etc.); in fact the need for calcium is higher for teenagers than for any other age group. Boys need about 1,000mg a day; girls need 800mg. This can be supplied by a glass of semi-skimmed milk, a pot of yoghurt and some broccoli. For girls calcium is important because if they don't build up their calcium reserves now, they may suffer from osteoporosis in later life. Girls also need more iron once they start menstruating (this is found especially in red meat, but also in fortified breakfast cereals, green vegetables and dried fruit). Vitamin C is also essential for iron absorption.

Establishing good eating habits

Eating is something your child will need to do for the rest of his or her life, and establishing good eating habits must be the primary aim of every parent. And by this I mean tasting, liking and enjoying good, fresh food. I have seen children who have not been introduced early enough, and by the time they get to school age they are resistant to anything new and will only eat plain pasta or chips (not that they get those often at St Peter's). We may have lost two generations to fatty and processed foods, who do not know how to buy, cook and eat well, but we can change this. To do it we need to establish good eating habits virtually from the cradle.

Introducing taste

I made many suggestions for baby foods in my first book, so I won't go into too much detail here, although I think it's a very important subject. Children need solid food from about six months (as well as their milk). It has been found that children who aren't introduced to solid food until after the age of nine months are more likely to turn into fussy eaters.

Needless to say, I advocate freshly cooked, sugar- and salt-free vegetable and fruit purées at first. Do this very gradually, one teaspoon per mealtime at first, and be patient: if at first you don't succeed, just try again, and again . . . Follow these first purées with blended food that is gradually less smooth, because babies also need to learn about texture (one of the elements of 'taste'). If they learn about texture as early as possible, they're less likely to reject textured foods later on. (I've seen school-age children being physically sick because a pot of fruit yoghurt has 'bits' in it.) Texture is also important because children have to learn to chew.

Puréed vegetables, such as carrots or peas, are important too, for their colour (another perceived element of 'taste'), their flavours, and for variety. Research at Birmingham University revealed that babies weaned on a diet of colourless, bland foods such as rusks, processed baby foods and milk are more likely to go on to prefer 'beige' carbohydrates such as crisps, white bread and chips (junk food in other words). It's all to do with a 'visual prototype', a preference for foods that are familiar. Children tend to reject foods that do not match the prototype, without even tasting them, which sets the pattern for future preferences. So if you feed your baby broccoli and carrots, even Brussels sprouts, he or she will probably continue eating them through childhood and adulthood.

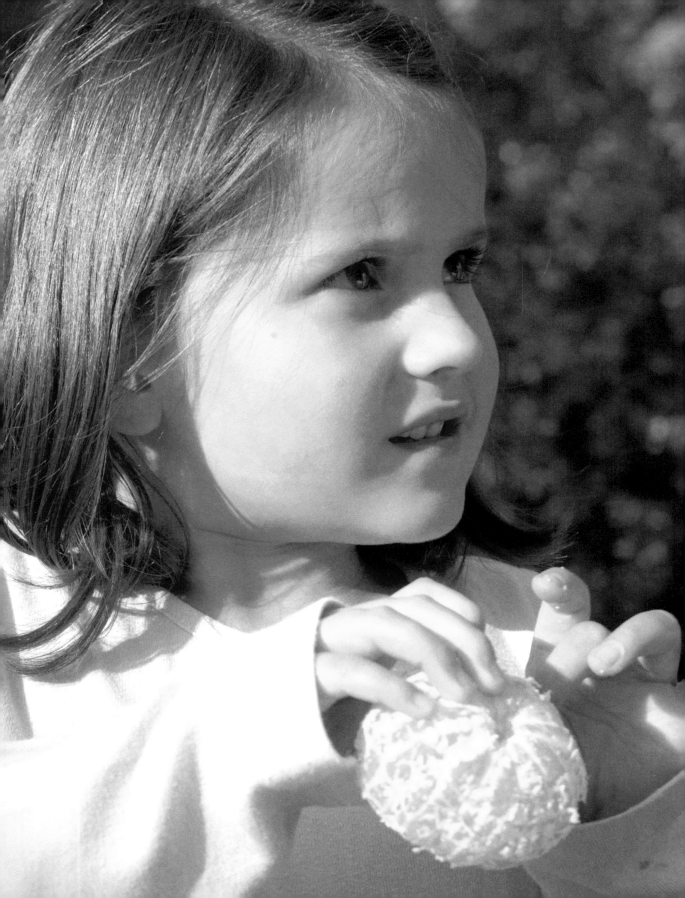

But why do the majority of us give babies bland foods? I think parents worry about what foods are safe for babies, and possibly feel that food out of a jar or packet is the safer option. This is a powerful argument for buying fresh, local, seasonal and organic: if you know where the broccoli was grown, that it is truly fresh and that it has not been sprayed, then you will probably be a lot happier cooking it for your baby.

Variety expands a baby's taste-buds. The more receptive he is to new tastes, the more likely an older child will be willing to eat different foods later in life. But if you find something your baby likes, don't feed it to him or her endlessly. I did this with my son Gareth when I discovered he liked fish. He had it for about three months, and doesn't much like fish now. I wonder why?

Pre-school children

This is the time when you can have most influence on what your children eat. Even if you are working and you have a childminder, nanny or doting grandmother looking after your child, you can still ask them to follow your healthy eating principles. It's different if your child goes to a day nursery (see page 93).

You are in charge. Nominally, though, because these can be the most problematic years for many parents: I'm thinking about the phrases 'terrible twos' and 'troublesome toddlers'. In general, babies aim to please you, but between the ages of about 18 months and four years, children become aware of relationships and of their own innate 'power'. This can cause difficulties, particularly at bedtime and at mealtimes. There can be a battle of wills, which all too often involves food: impatience and worry on the part of the parent (is he getting enough to eat?) and petulance and tantrums from the child. Here are a few stratagems.

● Sit down to eat with young (and older) children. They get used to the fact that mealtimes can be sociable occasions, and that food is a pleasure. Also if you, or others, are eating as well, he or she will get the idea.

● Give small portions, and make the food look attractive on the plate. A toddler might take one bite of a whole apple, but if you cut it up into smaller pieces he or she could well eat the lot.

● Let your child feed himself, even if it does mean a mess on the high-chair tray or table, and on the floor. This is all part of the learning process.

● Never say too much about the food – just put it in front of your child without comment. If you are matter-of-fact about it, food won't become an issue.

● Don't try to bribe: 'Eat your peas or you won't get any pudding', or 'If you don't eat your broccoli, you can't play on your bike.' This suggests that other things (pudding or playing) are nicer or more fun than eating vegetables.

● If a toddler won't eat something you put in front of him or her, or takes a long time, do not make a fuss. Get on with something else – the washing-up, or reading the paper.

● Not eating could be to do with craving attention. If you ignore difficult eating behaviour, your child will soon realize that attention and praise will follow eating rather than not eating.

● Don't offer an alternative food: they either eat it or they don't. It maddens me the number of parents who prepare not just one meal in the evening, but sometimes up to four, to accommodate everyone's different tastes!

● Never have a row about food. Losing your temper is a sign of weakness, and children recognize this and exploit it. Most children learn quickly that if they refuse to eat for long enough, adults will give in. And that's a dangerous precedent to set.

● Talk to your children, about what they like and don't like to eat, and why. Then there can be some sort of agreement: 'If you really don't like peppers, then I won't give them to you'. At least your child might feel you were more on his food wavelength.

● A child might not be hungry at mealtimes because he has had too many snacks. Pre-school children have small stomachs, so feeding them little and often is not totally forbidden, but avoid snacks too near to lunch or supper. And make those snacks nutritious – they need nutrient- and calorie-dense foods to help them grow.

● If you or someone else in the family doesn't like a food, either don't serve it or, if you do, don't let a fussy eater see that it's not particularly appreciated. Set a good example.

CHILDREN IN DAY NURSERY

A huge number of pre-school children go to nurseries, of which there are some 37,000 in Britain. If they are there all day, Monday to Friday, then virtually all they eat during the week comes from the nursery. If the quality of the food is poor, then children are getting a raw deal, for nursery food matters at least as much, if not more, than the food served in schools. Ask about meals when you are choosing a nursery. Their teeth need looking after too, something that has been addressed by a campaign aimed at nursery schools, Stop the Rot. Its initiator, Graham Wilding, a Lancashire dentist, says he sees too many children aged three or four with tooth decay. Participating nurseries now serve fruit instead of biscuits, ban chocolate and sweets, and get the children to brush their teeth after meals. That sounds like a good start to me.

The provision of nursery food is a concern to education officials in Scotland, and a consultation document, *Nutritional Guidance for Early Years*, was published at the beginning of 2005 to encourage good eating. (This document builds on Scotland's Hungry for Success scheme, which is working to transform the country's school meals.) I think we need something similar in England, but because most nursery provision is private, the Government may not get involved, as they only make funds available for state providers. Perhaps this could be my next campaign…

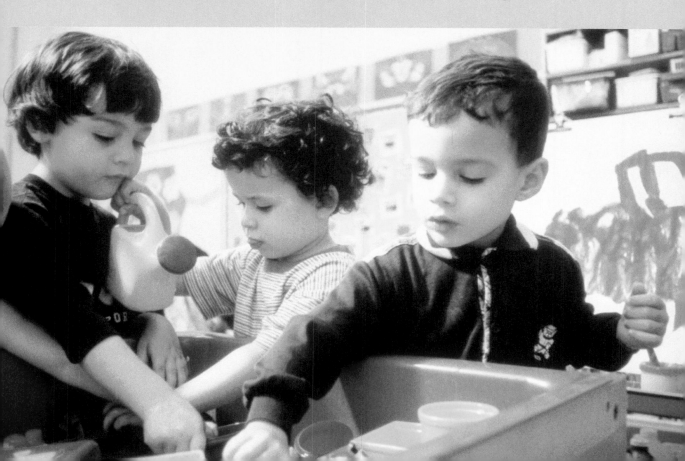

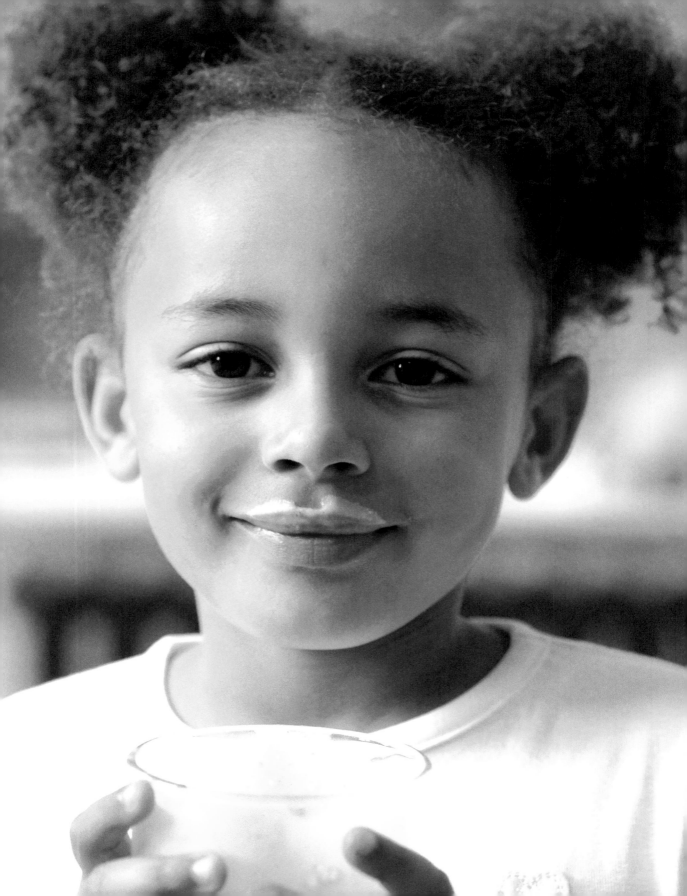

Children at primary school

It is when a child goes to school that established dietary patterns are most likely to change. For a start, this may be the first time someone other than you might be feeding your child – a dinner lady, for instance! Also, your child might be presented with choice for the first time, which can be very exciting. They are in charge of what they eat, not you. Peer pressure begins too. When I was at St Peter's, if one child came in and asked for a baked potato, we always noticed that eight others behind him would ask for the same. Similarly, if a child said he didn't like something, eight others behind him would say, 'Oh, I don't like that either.' Peer pressure is very powerful at this stage.

Protein foods and carbohydrates are important for when energy is needed straight away, but children need complex carbohydrates (see page 79), not crisps and biscuits which are high in calories but contain few nutrients, and often reduce children's appetite for healthier foods. It used to drive me mad – as it must a lot of dinner ladies – seeing the crisps and biscuits that children ate at break time at 10.30–10.45: of course they weren't hungry for their lunch at 11.45. That was before the School Fruit Scheme, though . . .

Children at school are often given money with which to buy their own lunch. This they spend as they like, often on the things you don't want them to have: fizzy drinks, sweets and biscuits in the school tuck shop or canteen, or chips on the way home. It infuriates me that some parents give their child a packed lunch because they are reluctant to spend under £2 on a meal that would see their child happily through the day. Yet they give in to peer pressure and fashion, and spend £80 on a pair of trainers or jeans (which will be outgrown quite soon anyway).

Older children

You know by now what I think children should be eating – fresh foods rather than processed – but it can be as difficult to get pubescent and teenage children to eat properly as it is a two-year-old. A survey published in 2004 found that the favourite brand of cuisine of 13- to 17-year-olds was McDonald's, followed by products from Cadbury, Pizza Hut, KFC and Coca-Cola. The trouble is that once they are at school, and have gained some sort of independence, your influence as a parent diminishes further, and that of their peers increases. They want to rebel, and turning away from the healthy food you have been giving them is one way of doing that. It's almost as if healthy food were uncool. All I can say in this situation is keep healthy foods at home: teenagers are continually hungry, and an apple or a couple of plums will be better

FOOD AND BEHAVIOUR

From my seventeen years or so of working with children, I believe there is a definite connection between food and children's behaviour, and although this is only anecdotal, do we really need to have everything explained by science? What has happened to good old common sense?

There is mounting evidence – from parents, teachers, nutritionists and doctors – that sugar- and fat-rich foods and a shortage of fresh foods are linked to ill-discipline, disruption and a growth in the numbers of children described as 'hyperactive', or diagnosed with attention deficit disorders. In the summer term of 2003, over 16,000 children were suspended for assault (on teachers and other pupils). Every day ten children are excluded for poor behaviour. No wonder then that this decline in classroom behaviour is of concern. The Government is promising a new 'culture of respect' and 'zero tolerance' of disruption in schools. I think good food, which

contains all the nutrients we need, should be the backbone of preventative health is schools.

Were there anti-social behaviour orders (ASBOs) in the 1950s? Are our children getting worse, and if they are, why? During my travels, working with schools all over the country, I met Megan Robinson, head teacher at Crondall Primary School in Hampshire. This school has taken on Food for Life targets, and since they have been serving fresh, local, seasonal and organic food, they have seen an improvement in the children's concentration and found them to be more alert in the afternoons. The same was also noted by Steve Armstrong, head teacher at Oakview Special School in Essex. I worked alongside the catering staff in this school, and must admit I was slightly apprehensive as to how the children would cope with the change. To my amazement, on the first day, they were queuing up for more. The teachers reported a calmer

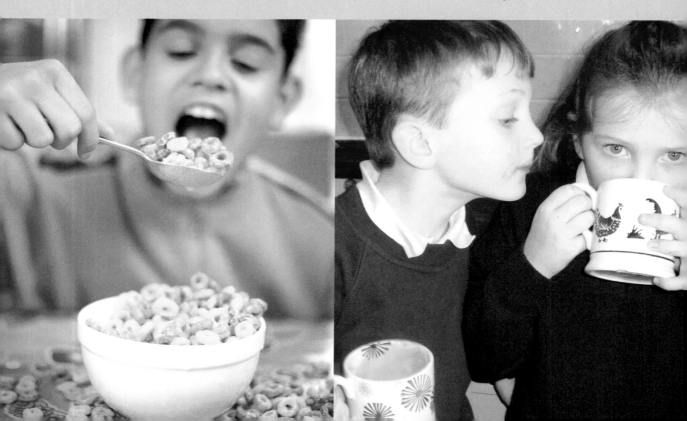

atmosphere, with the children being more receptive to learning. A growing band of head teachers are echoing these findings. A school in Norfolk that banned fizzy drinks three years ago noticed that attendance levels rose to 91 per cent, and that the GCSE pass rate doubled. They can't *prove* that the ban had anything to do with this, but I think it tells its own story.

Patrick Holford, a nutritional therapist, contributed to a *Tonight with Trevor McDonald* TV series in 2005, about the eating habits of three teenage boys. The boys' diets were changed: processed foods and fizzy drinks were banned, and their parents were given lists of what the boys should eat. The change in their behaviour over the following weeks was a revelation. At the beginning of the programme, they were moody, aggressive, some would say typical teenagers; but they gradually became chatty, lively and sociable (and one boy's acne cleared up). So is all this processed food good for us? I think not.

So what can we do? What can you do? For a start, stop giving children foods laden with additives, refined sugars, processed fats and refined carbohydrates. Children today are reported to consume 30 times more soft drinks and 25 times more confectionery than children in the 1950s, a terrifying statistic. But what do these foods actually do to our children? There is no clear evidence, but many think stimulants, refined sugars, trans and hydrogenated fats can contribute to anxiety, cravings, insomnia, tiredness, poor concentration, mood swings, hyperactivity, aggression, panic attacks, weight gain, depression, anti-social behaviour, asthma and other allergies.

As you read this, you can see how difficult it is for parents to be sure what to feed children. We're getting very mixed messages, and we need a clearer understanding of what is in our food. Should the Government put the brake on the food industry, and attempt to control what goes into our food? But maybe the answer is, simply, that we should all be eating fresh, home-cooked food. After all, what have we got to lose?

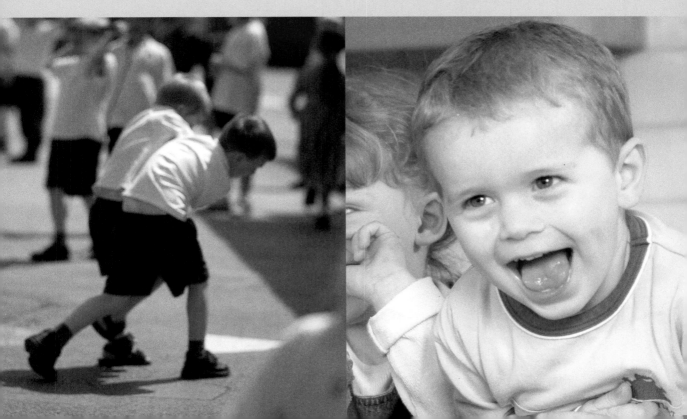

than nothing. Ensuring they have a good breakfast before school is one way of retaining a little control.

If your teenage child is fat because of this type of diet, it may be worrying for you. But don't harp on it, or make jokes, as this could diminish his or her self-esteem – very fragile at this stage – and lead to an eating disorder. There are no national statistics, only estimates, but it has been reported that as many as one in 50 young people may be affected by eating disorders. Anorexia mostly hits them between 14 and 18; bulimia generally comes later, between 18 and 25, when they leave the family home.

Some teenagers go the other way, and experiment with vegetarianism as their way of adopting an extra-healthy diet. If this happens to your child, ensure that they do not miss out on vital nutrients. Get a good nutrition book, and keep a variety of vegetables, fruit, grains, nuts and seeds at home – and perhaps consider offering a multivitamin supplement.

Perhaps you could encourage your teens to return to good eating habits by telling them about 'brain foods'. According to a piece in the Sunday Telegraph in May 2005, certain foods thought to feed and boost the brain were flying off supermarket shelves in the run-up to GCSEs, A-levels and university finals. Sales of salmon, tuna, avocado and blueberries apparently rocketed! But eating a can of sardines the night before an exam won't help: a healthy brain with maximum concentration powers relies on much more than a quick fix. A healthy diet from babyhood to adulthood is what optimizes brain function.

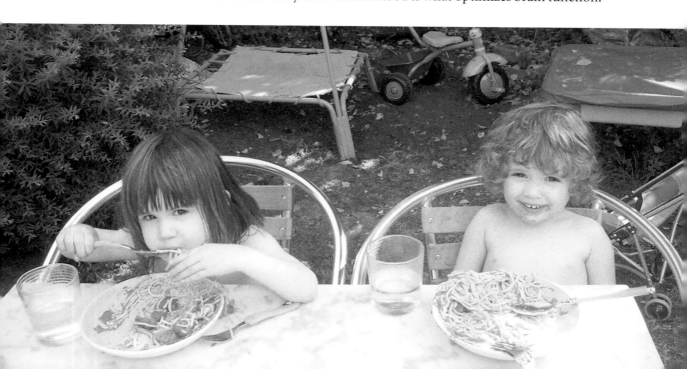

Eating together

There has been a huge social change in the last two generations. In the 1950s and 60s, when I was a child, most families sat down to eat together five or six times a week. We certainly did at home, and Sunday lunch, with both sets of grandparents, was sacrosanct. Nowadays, though, for a variety of reasons, only about one-third of parents eat with their children every day. A survey of over 2,000 parents (on the raisingkids.co.uk website) found that only 20 per cent of British families sat down to eat together once a week, sometimes even less.

Eating in

Why don't families eat together? Increasing time pressure on parents is one factor. A working father may come home too late to eat with his children, and has to eat later. My husband worked shifts at one point and I found it very difficult for us all to sit down at the same time some weeks. Working parents might have to rely on a child carer to give the children their supper in the evening, or may leave something in the fridge for older kids. A mother might feed young children early, while she and her partner sit down to eat after the children's bedtime. This also raises the question of what the children might be getting to eat: are they having 'children's' food, while she prepares 'proper' food for later? This idea of separate mealtimes for children is peculiarly British. They don't do it in France or Italy, where children are included in every meal, however late. (Perhaps our ideas in this country about children's bedtimes need rethinking.)

Television is another factor: the TV dinner (see page 49) really has had an effect on families eating together, as has the proliferation of TV channels, many of them aimed at children. Many families now eat, plates on their knees, in front of the flickering screen, which is not what I would call 'sociable'. Worse still, some children eat their meals separately in their bedrooms, glued to their favourite television programme, or munch while playing computer games. Central heating, perhaps surprisingly, has contributed to this latter phenomenon. Before its arrival, bedrooms were too cold for children to spend time in other than sleeping, and the whole family would remain together in the kitchen, usually the warmest room in the house. But many houses now have no room for a table, let alone a dining room, which has further 'eaten' into the concept of family meals.

Convenience or 'fast' food is the major contributor to fractured family mealtimes, I think. Quite apart from the takeaways that so many people rely on, supermarket ready meals are widely available, and can be popped in a microwave by any member of the family. This – what Joanna Blythman calls 'staggered eating' – tolls a death knell for family meals. (Ready meals are expensive too.)

I truly do believe that the family that eats together stays together. Sitting round a table, sharing a home-cooked meal, is one of the best ways possible of relating to one another. It's the ideal opportunity to exchange views, to air problems, to hear about each other's days, to laugh. If we are time-poor in other ways, then this is when we could be time-rich. Getting children to realize that eating is a pleasure is a huge step for their future sociability. They are also more likely to accept the food that is put in front of them, a very important factor when you have 'picky' eaters.

Research has also shown that children who had frequent family dinners ate some 40 per cent less fat and over 50 per cent more fruit and vegetables than those who ate separately. American research (from the School of Public Health) has found that increased family-meal frequency was associated, in adolescents, with reduced alcohol, tobacco and marijuana use, as well as a whole range of other psychological and social benefits (increased self-esteem, for a start). The conclusion of the research was that family meals were a sign of family closeness, which can't be a bad thing.

my favorit meal is a roast diner.

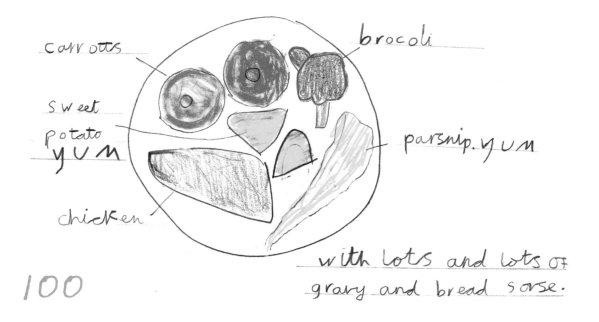

carrotts

brocoli

sweet potato yum

parsnip. yum

chicken

with lots and lots of gravy and bread sorse.

Eating out

Once, eating out was a rare treat. Our family ate out only occasionally when I was young, to celebrate something like a birthday. Now, because we as a nation have more disposable income, we eat out a lot more. Although I love eating with my family at home, I also enjoy eating out with them (it means I don't have to cook!).

Children should be included in trips to restaurants. It's another part of their food education, introducing them to new experiences, to new sights, sounds, attitudes and tastes – as well as to which knife and fork to use for each course. But in Britain we seem to be reticent about this, much more so than on the Continent. Restaurants in France and Italy, for example, welcome children, fussing over them, looking after them. Here, taking children to a restaurant can be fraught. For a start more than a few restaurants have a 'no children' policy, which I think is appalling. It's as if children are regarded as being a separate species. I know other people's badly behaved children can be a nightmare in a restaurant, but eating out can also be the prime time when children behave well, enjoying being treated as adults.

A few months ago I was in a local restaurant when a family came in – parents, grandparents and two young children armed with colouring books and crayons. They ordered their meal: one of the children ordered risotto, the other game (to my surprise). On the next table two adults got up, went to the manager and complained, saying that had they known the restaurant allowed children they would not have booked a table. I was incensed. Here were two well-behaved children: what could they possibly complain about? And how are children supposed to learn about food and eating out if they are not allowed in a good restaurant? It's beyond me.

Far too often, rather than face attitudes such as these, parents choose to take their children to a restaurant with a 'child-friendly' menu – generally chicken nuggets and chips, burgers and chips, or sausage and chips. But why, oh why should we allow this to be the norm? And why do so many eating places, good restaurants among them, have specific menus for children? When we take children out, there is no reason why they shouldn't eat the same food as adults, just smaller portions (or an adult portion divided in two, on two plates, for two children). This would be a much better solution, but it calls for education – for restaurants, for parents and for children. Maybe the answer is to only go to restaurants that will provide small portions for children, and avoid those with dull children's menus. They would eventually get the message . . .

AND TO DRINK?

Water

The only liquid we need is water. That goes for children too, once they have been weaned off breast (or formula) milk. Breast milk is quite sweet, though, and children's innate tendency towards sweetness has been exploited by drink manufacturers. But children don't need sweet drinks, or drinks stuffed full of gases, additives, E-numbers and caffeine. More importantly these drinks are thought to contribute to obesity, behavioural problems, and lack of concentration.

Water should be offered from the very beginning (boiled and cooled for babies). Some 70 per cent of our body weight consists of water, and adults should drink 2.5 litres (4$^1/_2$ pints) a day, children about 500ml (a scant pint). Even the mildest dehydration can cause constipation, headache, irritability and lack of concentration. I'm pleased that water is now allowed in classrooms, and that water is provided by schools at lunchtime and in the playground.

Tap water is fine, I think. Its bacterial and chemical composition is subject to very strict regulation, and it is far cheaper than bottled waters (which are up to 700 times more expensive). Tap water can taste, though, of chlorine at times, just dead at others. If you are concerned you can use a water filter. Keep a 2 litre (4 pint) bottle of tap water in the fridge – chilling somehow enlivens flavour – or serve it with lots of ice, or fresh herbs (mint is good) encased in ice cubes, or slices of lemon or lime, perhaps even a curly straw. Make water look attractive, and children won't be tempted in other directions. At the simplest, just don't offer alternatives.

Milk and other drinks

To me, milk is a food rather than a drink. Children need to have a fair proportion of it for its calcium content: children under five will need about 600ml (1 pint) a day; from 11 to 18, because of the pubertal growth spurt, calcium requirements double (see page 88) so they need about 900ml (1$^1/_2$ pints). Babies under two should have full-fat milk, thereafter you can try semi-skimmed; organic is best (see page 28). If your child doesn't like to drink milk, offer milk puddings, white and other sauces, smoothies, and milkshakes (see pages 108–9). You can serve milk hot in a chocolate, cocoa or similar drink (although some of these are full of sugar).

Fruit drinks and fruit squashes can be packed full of sugar and other additives – even sugar-free varieties – so are best avoided. Some supposed 'fruit' drinks contain as little as 12–15 per cent real fruit: just imagine what the rest is. Freshly squeezed citrus and other juices are fine as an occasional treat with meals. They provide Vitamin C which aids iron absorption. Juicing somehow intensifies the sugars, though; perhaps dilute them with water to reduce the acidic taste as well as the acidity that can eat into tooth enamel. If you are lucky enough to have a juicer, play around with vegetable and fruit combinations – pear and carrot, tomato and orange etc. The kids could help with this or even invent their own.

Children should not have drinks like tea and coffee as they contain tannins which interfere with iron absorption. Older children might enjoy herbal teas, which taste good.

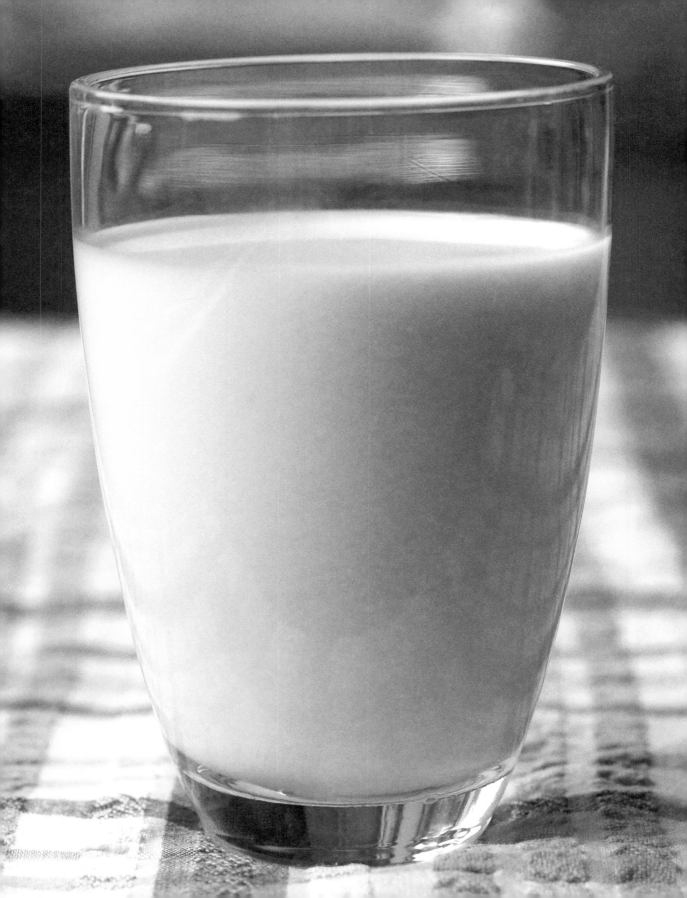

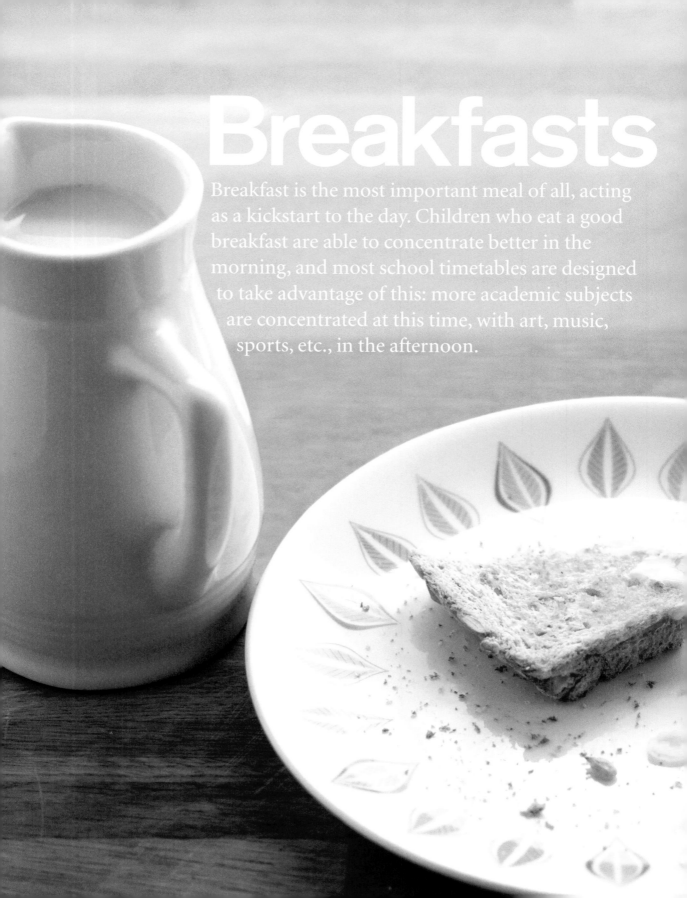

Breakfasts

Breakfast is the most important meal of all, acting as a kickstart to the day. Children who eat a good breakfast are able to concentrate better in the morning, and most school timetables are designed to take advantage of this: more academic subjects are concentrated at this time, with art, music, sports, etc., in the afternoon.

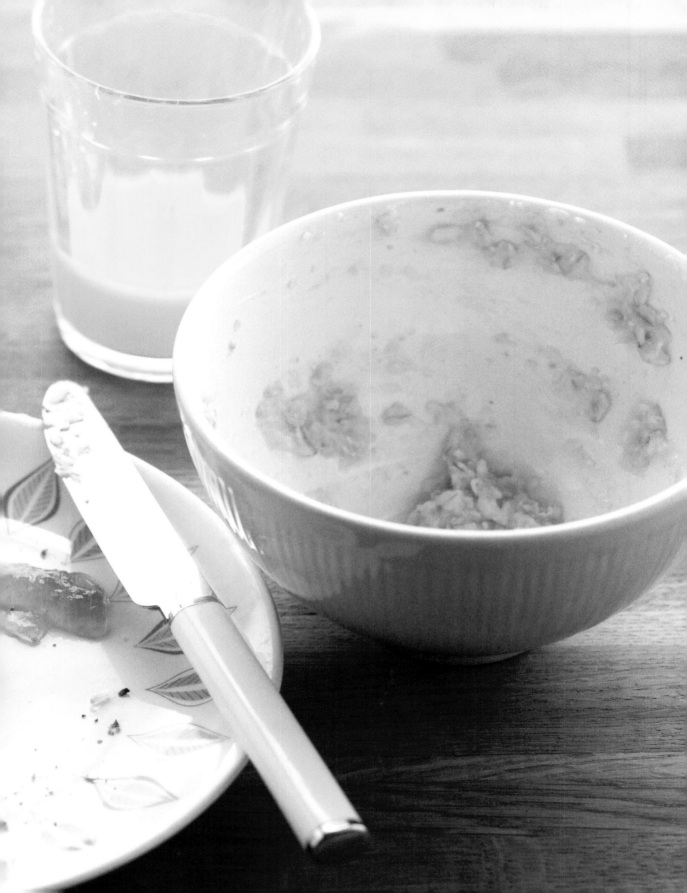

IF CHILDREN DO NOT have a good breakfast, their reading, writing and number work can suffer. Many schools are now offering breakfast clubs to cater for children whose parents go to work early and have no time to prepare breakfast. In theory this is an excellent idea, but most only offer cereal and toast (which is easy enough to prepare at home). But is this putting extra pressure on dinner ladies and teaching staff? Who is doing the doling out of breakfasts, who is supervising the children and who is paying for all this?

Children are hungry in the morning after a night's fast, so breakfast should consist of something substantial, which is full of nutrients. Cereal and milk are very good, but make sure the cereal isn't too processed. Muesli and porridge (see pages 115 and 112) are best. Natural bio-live yoghurt with some chopped or soft fruit is nutritious; toast some seeds (pumpkin, sunflower, sesame) and scatter them on top for extra flavour and crunch. Dried fruit is also very good, and the compote on page 113 (as well as the stewed apples with blueberries on page 261) could be prepared the night before, to be eaten cold in the morning. A yoghurt smoothie or milky fruity drink is excellent, and takes only moments to prepare in a blender. Children also love toast, butter and jam or marmalade. You can try all sorts of different breads, or think about muffins (bought or home-made), bagels, crispbreads, etc.

At the weekend you will have more time, and this is when breakfast could be cooked: at its simplest, a boiled or poached egg, or any of the recipes which follow. Eggs are full of protein; always choose organic free-range if at all possible. Scrambled eggs, for instance, can be varied in a number of ways: with spices as on page 122, simply with chopped fresh chives on top, or (for a very special occasion) some slivers of smoked salmon. Fishcakes or vegetable burgers might be an idea, or my bubble and squeak (see pages 167, 177 and 196), served with grilled tomatoes or mushrooms or bacon (good for high tea or supper as well). The smoked haddock pancakes on page 162 make a good celebratory breakfast: a friend serves this at Christmas.

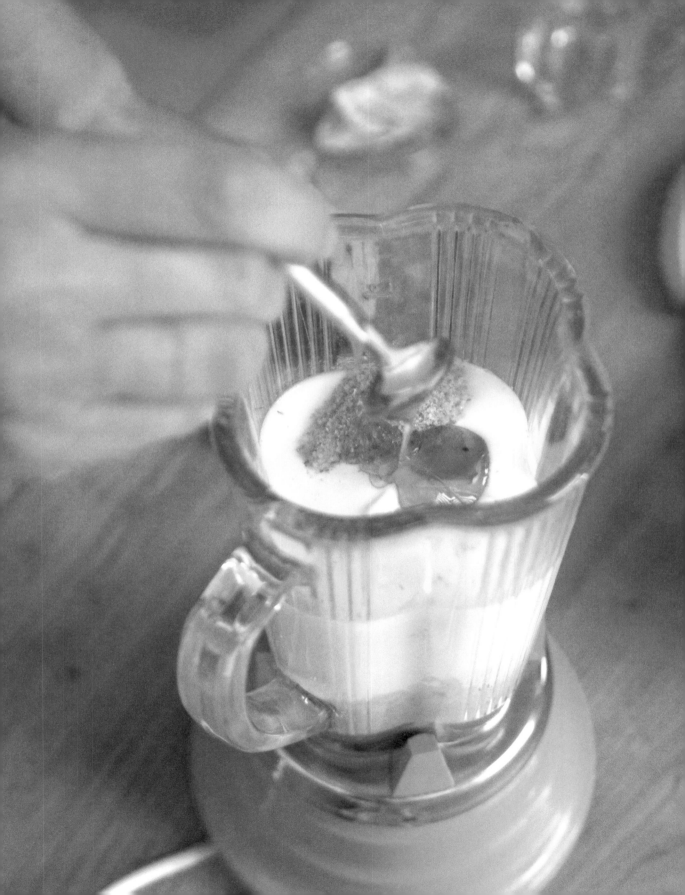

Smoothies

Breakfast in a glass. This is a great way for children to have plenty of fresh fruit, and the combinations are endless. The children can also make these on their own, so just stand back and let them experiment. Other fruits they could use include melon, pineapple, pawpaw, peaches, nectarines, ripe pears and apricots.

Banana smoothie

SERVES 4

4 large bananas, peeled and roughly chopped
2 tablespoons natural bio-live yoghurt
250ml (9fl oz) cold semi-skimmed milk
1 teaspoon runny honey
1 tablespoon wheatgerm
¼ teaspoon ground cinnamon (optional)

● Put the bananas in the blender. Add the yoghurt and milk, and blend until smooth. Add the honey, wheatgerm and cinnamon, and blend again for 5–10 seconds.

● Pour into glasses and serve immediately.

Strawberry/raspberry/mango smoothie

● Use 250g (9oz) strawberries or raspberries or peeled chopped mango, instead of the banana.

Fruit and berry smoothie

● Use a combination of any fruit and some berries – made up to the 250g (9oz) weight – instead of the banana.

Innocent mango, pineapple and banana fresh fruit smoothie

The nice people at Innocent, who manufacture healthy drinks, have designed a one-off recipe for this book.

Their smoothies are made by mixing whole crushed fruit with fresh fruit juices, which means that you get more of the fruit into the drink. In fact, each 85g (3oz) of crushed fruit equals one portion of fruit, helping your kids towards their sacred 'five a day' (see page 82). Smoothies simply provide more of the vitamins, minerals and fibre, by virtue of the fact they contain all of that squashed-up fruit. So dig out your juicers and blenders and get on with it!

MAKES about 1 litre (1¾ pints)

1 juicy mango, peeled and sliced
½ pineapple, peeled and cored
1 banana, peeled and roughly
    chopped
juice of 2 oranges
juice of ½ lime
juice of 2 apples

● Put the prepared mango, pineapple and banana into the blender.

● Add the juice of the oranges: use a citrus press or just add about 100ml (3½ fl oz) bought freshly squeezed orange juice. Add the lime and apple juices: for the latter, use a centrifugal juicer or instead add about 100ml (3½ fl oz) bought pure apple juice (stay away from concentrated juice).

● Put the lid on the blender, and blend until the desired consistency is achieved.

Variations

Why not try different combinations of fruits? There aren't any rules to making a smoothie, but here are some useful tips.

● Wash your fruit before you use it.

● Chill fruit in the fridge beforehand to get ice-cold smoothies.

● Vary the fruits you use as much as you like, trying to stick to those in season.

● Banana adds sweetness and texture to a smoothie.

● Apple juice adds sweetness to sharp fruits.

● Orange juice (or a squeeze of lemon) brings out the fruitiness and adds a nice citrus zing.

● Add some natural yoghurt if you want to boost calcium intake.

● Use a mixture of juice and whole crushed fruit to get the right texture.

● Always serve and drink your smoothie straight away.

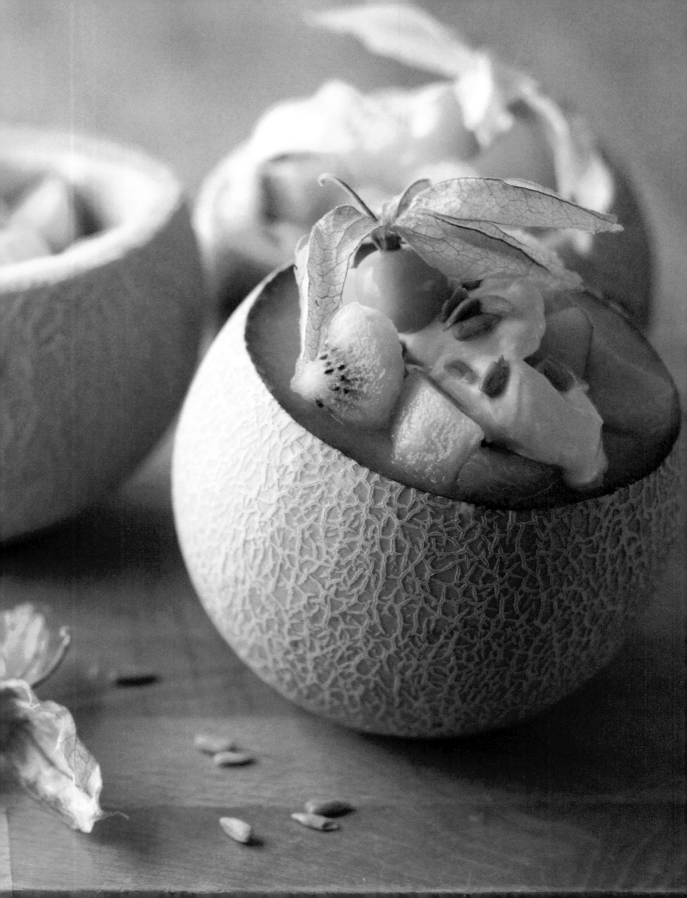

Fruit-stuffed melon cups

We are told to eat five portions of fruit and vegetables every day, and this recipe – which is good for breakfast or a pudding – just about fits the bill. The fruit used below is a guide; you can decide what to put in the cups. But I know that children love this, both the tastes and the unusual container.

SERVES 4

2 galia melons, halved widthways and deseeded
4 oranges, peeled and segmented
4 kiwi fruit, peeled
4 pears, peeled and segmented
300ml (10fl oz) orange juice
4 tablespoons natural bio-live yoghurt
1 teaspoon sunflower seeds
8 Cape gooseberries (physalis)

● Scoop the flesh out of the melon halves, leaving the shells, which you are going to use as bowls.

● Cut all the fruit (including the melon flesh, but not the gooseberries) into small bite-sized pieces and mix together in a large bowl. Pour in the orange juice, mix, and pile into the melon shells.

● Place a tablespoon of yoghurt in the centre and sprinkle with the sunflower seeds. Finish with two Cape gooseberries per melon shell.

Fruity porridge

If you are using oatmeal rather than rolled or flaked oats, you can start this the night before. You can also cook the fruit the night before. Try using 225g (8oz) strawberries or raspberries, or 2 bananas with 55g (2oz) raisins and 1 tablespoon honey, or 1 ripe peach or nectarine with 115g (4oz) raspberries.

SERVES 4

200g (7oz) oatmeal or rolled or flaked oats
1 litre (1¾ pints) semi-skimmed milk
225g (8oz) blackberries or blueberries, washed
1 apple, peeled, cored and sliced
1 tablespoon soft brown sugar

● Place the oatmeal in a saucepan with the milk and leave to soak overnight. The rolled or flaked oats do not need soaking.

● Place the blackberries in a saucepan with the apple slices and 50ml (2fl oz) water. Simmer for about 10 minutes until soft. Add the sugar, remove from the heat and leave to cool.

● To cook the porridge, slowly bring the milk and oats to the boil, stirring all the time, then cook, still stirring (porridge tends to catch on the base of the pan), for about 10–15 minutes until thick.

● Pour into bowls and add the fruit topping.

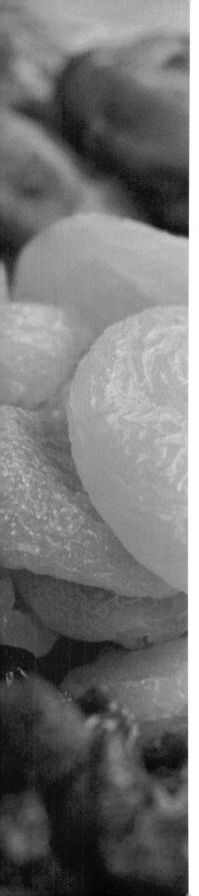

Dried fruit compote

When fruits are dried, their sweetness intensifies. You can buy organic dried fruit, which is preferable to fruit preserved with sulphur. Organic dried apricots are particularly delicious, dark in colour, with a toasted flavour. Most compotes use a sugar syrup, and of course you can add some, but I don't think it's necessary. Serve with natural bio-live yoghurt, and with some toasted seeds, hazelnuts or flaked almonds on top. It's delicious with the muesli on page 115, or with some good vanilla ice-cream.

SERVES 4

450g (1lb) mixed dried fruit, cut into bite-sized pieces (try apricots, figs, raisins, peaches, pears, dates, mango, pineapple, pawpaw, prunes, apple rings)
2–3 thin strips lemon or lime rind
a 1cm (½ in) piece stem ginger (optional)
1 cinnamon stick

● Before cutting dried fruit, wipe your knife with a bit of oiled kitchen paper. Just cover the fruit with cold water in a saucepan and leave to soak for a few hours, or overnight.

● Put the fruit pan on the heat, and add the lemon rind, ginger if using, and cinnamon. Bring to the boil, then reduce the heat, cover and simmer gently for about 20 minutes. The fruit should be tender, and the liquid reduced (it will thicken further in the fridge).

● Remove the lemon rind, ginger and cinnamon, and leave to cool. Serve chilled.

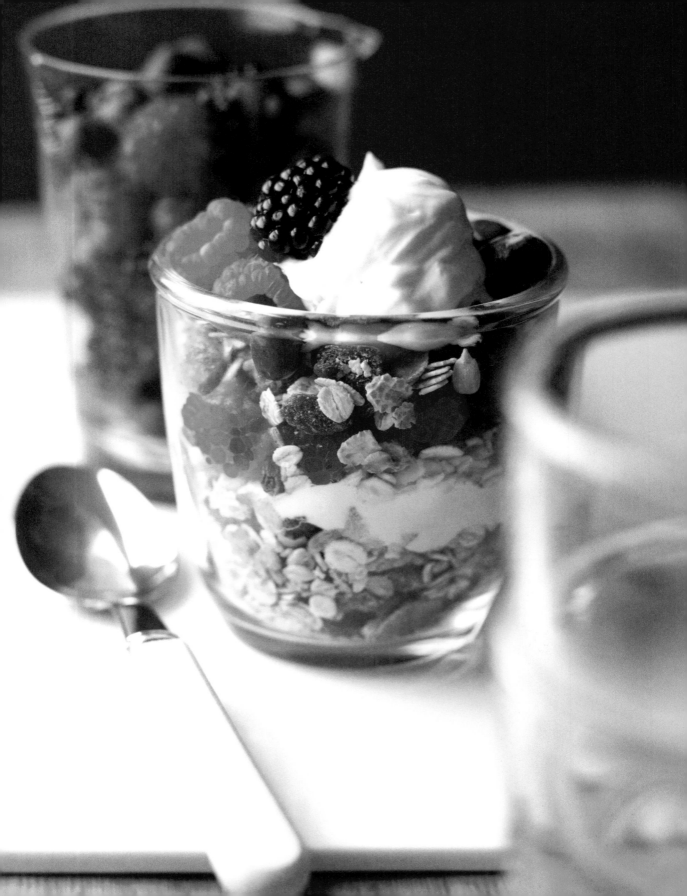

Home-made muesli

You can double the quantities of the different flakes and store the muesli in an airtight container for about 1 month. Just add the fruit when you are ready to serve.

MAKES ABOUT 350g (12oz)

225g (8oz) rolled oats
25g (1oz) wheatgerm
55g (2oz) oatmeal
25g (1oz) sunflower seeds
15g (½oz) pine nuts

● Mix all the ingredients together in a large bowl. Transfer to an airtight container and just use the quantity you need.

Variations

Try adding, per portion (55g/2oz):

● 15g (½oz) dried fruit, 1 tablespoon runny honey and 2 tablespoons natural bio-live yoghurt

● 1 banana, peeled and sliced, with 25g (1oz) strawberries and 2 tablespoons natural bio-live yoghurt

● 1 tablespoon Greek yoghurt, 1 teaspoon runny honey, 25g (1oz) each of green grapes and blueberries, or 25g (1oz) black grapes

● Anything and everything that is in season – let your imagination go!

French toast

Also known as 'eggy bread' – beloved of Girl Guides – and, I think, 'pain perdu' ('lost bread' in French), this is a quick hot dish to make for breakfast or tea. Use different types of bread, pre-cut with crusts off. If you want to make it savoury, you could use breads flavoured with cheese, sun-dried tomatoes or olives (good with grilled bacon). If you prefer the sweeter option, use fruit or nut breads, or some panettone (an Italian sweet cake-bread), and serve with honey and some cinnamon.

SERVES 4

4 slices bread, crusts cut off, cut into triangles
2 large eggs, beaten with 1 tablespoon milk
25g (1oz) butter

● Soak the slices of bread in the egg and milk for about 5 minutes.

● Heat half the butter in a frying pan, and fry half the bread triangles until golden on both sides. Cook the remaining triangles in the rest of the butter. Serve immediately.

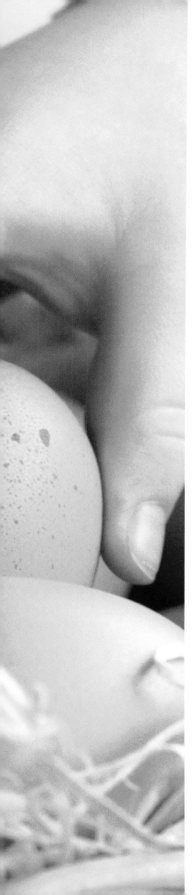

Tidgy English breakfast

This is basically a baked egg, but specially for breakfast, and it is very easy. There are many possible variations as well. You can bake them in any small ovenproof pots or ramekins, or in different types of container (see the following recipe). You can bake them plain, or put something tasty in the bottom of the dish as here: try some grated cheese, baked beans, leftover bits of cooked chicken or turkey, or chopped ham, some blanched peas or sweetcorn, chopped tomatoes, or a spoonful of cooked spinach. Warm these additions through in the dishes in the oven for about 10 minutes before adding the eggs. Try sprinkling some grated cheese on the top before baking.

SERVES 4

2 good-quality sausages
olive oil
4 rashers bacon
4 eggs

● Preheat the oven to 200°C/400°F/Gas 6.

● Cut the sausages into four pieces each, and gently fry in a little olive oil for about 10–15 minutes. Cut the bacon into strips, add to the sausage, and cook for a further 5–10 minutes.

● Lightly grease four ramekin dishes and place the sausage and bacon in the bottom. Carefully break an egg into each dish. Bake in the preheated oven until the eggs are set but still soft, about 5 minutes.

Tomato baked eggs

With this variant on the baked egg theme, the children can eat the container as well! This dish would be good for either breakfast or tea in the evening, served with bacon, a sausage perhaps, and some crusty bread or toast. You could put something underneath the egg (see page 117), and you could sprinkle some grated cheese on top before baking.

SERVES 4

4 medium beef tomatoes, washed
olive oil
4 large eggs
25g (1oz) Parmesan cheese, freshly grated (optional)
chopped fresh basil or parsley

● Preheat the oven to 180°C/350°F/Gas 4.

● Slice a lid off each beef tomato. Scrape out the seeds from the tomatoes to make 'containers'. Lightly oil an ovenproof dish and put the tomatoes in it. Bake in the preheated oven for about 5 minutes, then remove from the oven.

● Break an egg into each tomato container, top with cheese if you like – and the tomato lids, at an angle – and return to the oven for another 5 minutes. Serve immediately, with a sprinkle of chopped herb to decorate.

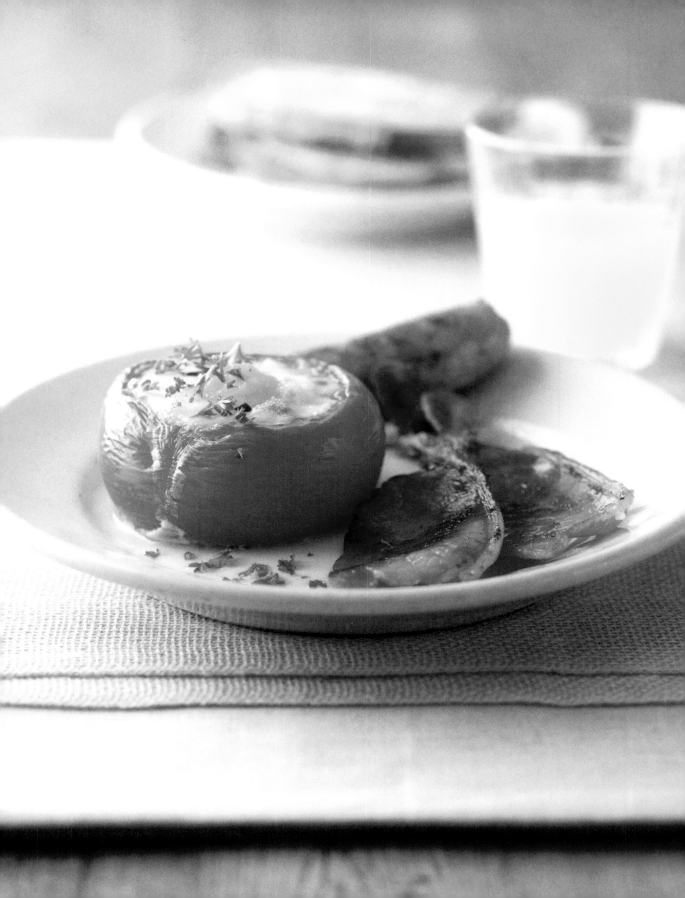

Open soufflé omelette

There is nothing better to my mind than really good eggs for a great start to the day. I have given the instructions for a soufflé omelette here, but you can just make a plain omelette, by whipping the egg whites and yolks together before continuing with the method as below. At the weekend, for a treat, try a special filling or topping, which you can make from anything you like.

SERVES 4

8 large eggs
½ teaspoon freshly ground black pepper
25g (1oz) butter

● Preheat the grill well.

● You will need two bowls. To separate the eggs, crack one at a time, and carefully tip the yolk from one half of the shell to the other, letting the white drop into one of the bowls. Put the yolk in the other bowl. Do the same for all the eggs.

● Whisk the yolks together well, and sprinkle with the pepper. Add flavourings at this stage if liked (see below). Whisk the whites until they are nearly doubled in size. Gradually add the whipped white to the yolk, folding in a figure of eight until all the white has been absorbed.

● In a large omelette pan, about 25cm (10in) in diameter, melt the butter until it is foaming but not brown. Add the egg mixture and cook over a medium heat for 1 minute, so that the egg begins to set at the bottom.

● Add your chosen topping (see below), and then place under a hot grill. Cook until the egg is just set on the top and bubbling around the edges. Remove and cool a little before cutting into four wedges.

Ideas for fillings/toppings

Mushroom Use 225g (8oz) mushrooms – button, flat, field, or more unusual ones like shiitake or chanterelles. Wash, dry and slice, and cook in a little butter for 3–5 minutes. Mix with 1 tablespoon crème fraîche, 25g (1oz) freshly grated Parmesan cheese, and a small grating of nutmeg. Put on top of the omelette before grilling.

Herb Add 1 teaspoon chopped fresh parsley, chives or chervil (or try a combination) to the egg yolks before mixing with the egg white. You could add a little cheese when putting under the grill (see below).

Cheese Use 115g (4oz) cheese. Grate Cheddar or Red Leicester on to the omelette before it goes under the grill.

Ham Put 225g (8oz) diced ham on to the omelette before it goes under the grill. You could also add halved cherry tomatoes.

Bacon Use 2 rashers per person. Remove the rind and cut the bacon into strips 1cm (½in) thick. Dry-fry until cooked, about 5–10 minutes. Add to the egg-yolk mixture (perhaps with some cherry tomatoes as above).

Potato and bacon Peel 115g (4oz) potatoes, and cut into small dice. Boil in water for about 5–8 minutes, then drain well. Using the omelette pan and the recipe butter, fry the potato dice until brown. Add 115g (4oz) cooked and chopped bacon, then pour the egg mixture into the pan and cook as above. Sprinkle some cheese on top if you like before grilling.

Potato and cheese Prepare the potatoes as above. Pour in the eggs, then top with 55g (2oz) grated cheese, and put under the grill to finish.

Salmon Cut 225g (8oz) salmon fillet into thin strips, and fry in a little extra butter for about 2–3 minutes. Mix with 2 tablespoons crème fraîche and a few chopped chives. Cook the omelette, then top with the salmon mixture and put under the grill.

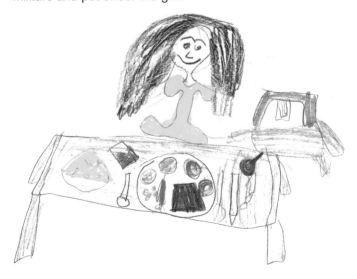

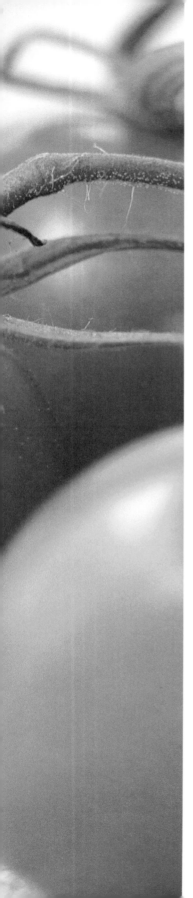

Mexican scrambled eggs

Scrambled eggs with a bit of a kick. If you handle chilli flakes, or fresh chilli, wash your hands very well, and never touch your eyes.

SERVES 4

3 tablespoons olive oil
8 spring onions, trimmed and roughly sliced
1 garlic clove, peeled and crushed
1 pinch chilli flakes
300g (10½oz) ripe tomatoes, deseeded and finely chopped
4 large eggs
2 tablespoons chopped fresh parsley

To serve
4 slices toast

● Heat the oil in a medium frying pan, and fry the spring onion, garlic, chilli flakes and tomato for about 8 minutes.

● Beat the eggs in a bowl, and stir with the parsley into the tomato mix.

● Cook, stirring, over a low heat until the egg is scrambled but still a bit wet. Pile on to toast and serve immediately.

Bacon and potato cakes

Serve these for breakfast with a poached egg on top, or for supper with a parsley sauce (see page 61) and some grilled tomatoes or flat field mushrooms.

SERVES 4

350g (12oz) unsmoked bacon, roughly chopped
1kg (2¼lb) potatoes, peeled and quartered
175g (6oz) onions, peeled and finely diced
olive oil
2 spring onions, sliced
1 tablespoon chopped fresh parsley
1 large egg, beaten
freshly ground black pepper

Suitable for freezing after shaping. Open freeze on a baking tray then pack into freezer bags.

● Dry-fry the chopped bacon until nearly crisp. Boil the potatoes for 20 minutes until just soft. Meanwhile, fry the onions in a little olive oil until soft and golden brown, about 5–10 minutes. Add the spring onions, and cook for a further minute. Cool.

● Drain the potatoes, and mash over a low heat until dry. Put the bacon in a large mixing bowl with the potato and onion, parsley, egg and black pepper. Mix well to incorporate the egg.

● Heat a large frying pan with 1–2 tablespoons oil. Using a large spoon, scoop about a tablespoon of mixture into the frying pan and flatten slightly with the back of the spoon to create a 'cake'. Continue to do this with the remaining mixture and cook on each side for 3–4 minutes or until golden brown. The mixture should make eight cakes.

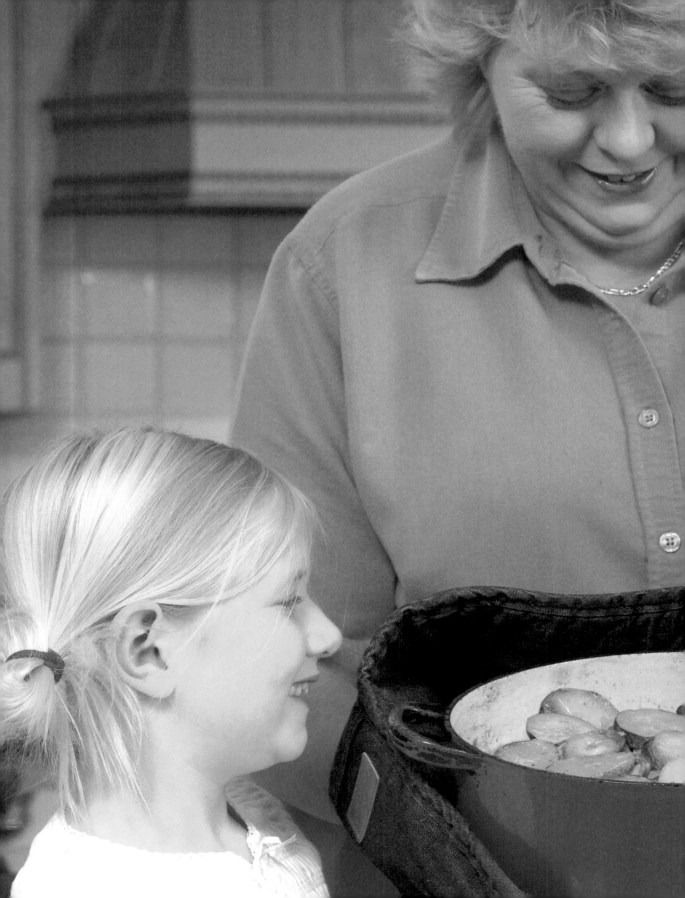

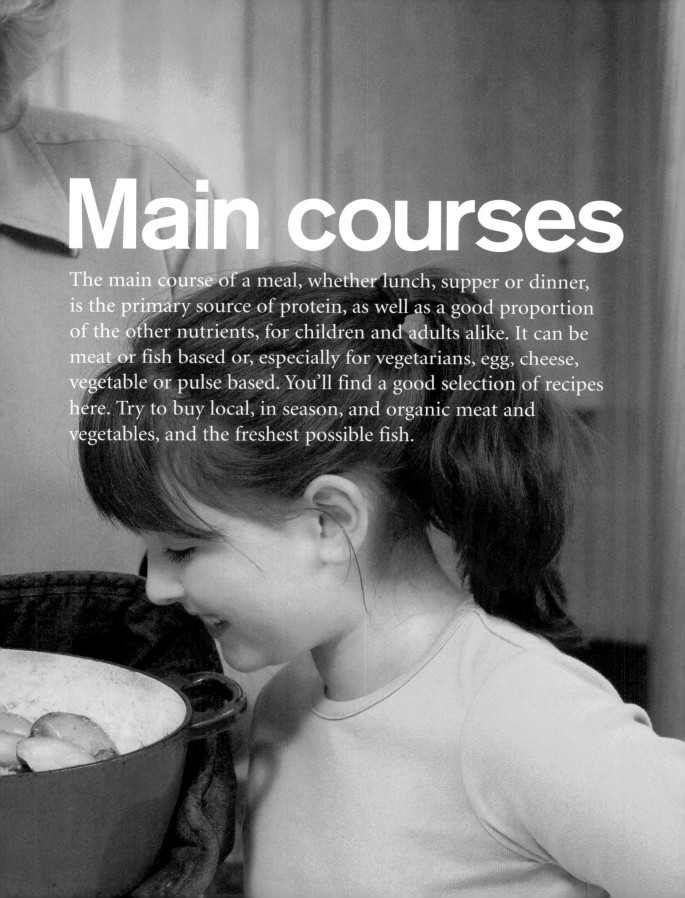

Main courses

The main course of a meal, whether lunch, supper or dinner, is the primary source of protein, as well as a good proportion of the other nutrients, for children and adults alike. It can be meat or fish based or, especially for vegetarians, egg, cheese, vegetable or pulse based. You'll find a good selection of recipes here. Try to buy local, in season, and organic meat and vegetables, and the freshest possible fish.

DINNER LADIES ARE most concerned with the main course. They want to feed their children adequately and healthily, knowing how beneficial this is to a child's work in the afternoon, but are also aware that they might be feeding a child who has had no breakfast, or who is going home to a ketchup sandwich or instant noodles in pots. But if dinner ladies sometimes don't know what children are eating at home, so some parents don't know what their children are getting at school (although this, thankfully, is becoming more a thing of the past). For if their child has not had a nutritious main course at school in the middle of the day, then the evening meal at home has to be packed full of nutrients to make up for it.

The recipes in this section are a mixture of flavours and influences, reflecting traditional British dishes as well as ideas from other cuisines/cultures that appeal to children. (We always want to introduce children to new tastes.) Meat, especially red meat, is important in a child's diet because it is a significant source of iron as well as other nutrients. Vegetables, which children can often be resistant to, are 'disguised' in many of the recipes, in the stew on page 136 for instance, and quite a few fruits are used as well. The sweetness in conjunction with meat appeals to children. Fish too is an important source of protein and other nutrients, and because it is easy to digest it's good to offer for an evening meal. There are quite a few ideas here that will appeal to children and they are cooked in a healthy way (baked instead of fried, for instance).

Children who don't eat fish or meat have to eat foods that, in combination, will supply the proper amounts of protein needed. Protein-rich foods include eggs (see Breakfasts for more ideas), cheese, milk, yoghurt, wheatgerm and soya. Pulses are good sources of protein (see the recipes here, and there are some in Vegetables and Salads), as are grains (rice, wheat, oats etc., and the produce made from them such as pasta, bread and cereals), nuts and seeds. However, these are mostly so-called incomplete proteins that need to be eaten in combination with other incomplete proteins, preferably at the same meal (for example, grains and pulses – beans on toast) to provide complete protein. Remember too you can combine complete proteins with incomplete – pasta with cheese, rice with vegetables and eggs, pastry with cheese and pulses, a pizza with a healthy topping (see Snacks, page 236, for more ideas).

meaty matters

Hamburger loaf

A meat loaf in other words, but with the magic word 'hamburger' attached …You could serve this with the tomato sauce on page 142, or onion gravy (see page 143).

SERVES 4

olive oil
1kg (2¼lb) minced pork
175g (6oz) wholemeal breadcrumbs
2 rashers bacon, rinded and chopped
115g (4oz) red onion, peeled and diced
55g (2oz) red pepper, deseeded and diced
1 teaspoon chopped fresh thyme
55g (2oz) pine kernels
1 egg, beaten

Suitable for freezing after cooking. Defrost then cover and warm in the oven (at the same temperature), until piping hot, about 20–25 minutes.

● Preheat the oven to 180°C/350°F/Gas 4. Lightly grease a 450g (1lb) loaf tin with olive oil.

● Put the minced pork and breadcrumbs in a large mixing bowl.

● Heat a little olive oil in a pan, add the bacon, onion and red pepper, and gently cook for 5–10 minutes until soft. Add to the pork and breadcrumbs in the mixing bowl along with the thyme and pine kernels, and combine well. Pour the egg over the meat mixture. Stir until everything is thoroughly mixed together.

● Press the mixture into the prepared tin. Cut a piece of greaseproof paper to fit the top and place over the loaf. Bake in the preheated oven for 40–45 minutes, taking the greaseproof paper off for the last 10 minutes.

Lancashire hotpot

This is great on a cold winter's day when the children come in from school. Serve with some crusty bread. Ask your butcher to dice the lamb for you; he might even core the kidneys for you. Kidneys are traditional in a hotpot, and I think it is good to introduce them to children, but leave them out if your children really don't like them.

SERVES 4

olive oil
1kg (2¼ lb) best end neck of lamb, diced
4 lambs' kidneys, cored and diced
225g (8oz) carrots, peeled and sliced
225g (8oz) parsnips, peeled and sliced
2 red onions, peeled and sliced
450g (1lb) potatoes, peeled and sliced
300ml (10fl oz) lamb stock (see page 223)
1 sprig fresh rosemary
25g (1oz) butter

● Preheat the oven to 180°C/350°F/Gas 4.

● In a pan heat a little olive oil and brown the diced lamb. Put the lamb and the kidneys in a casserole dish, then arrange the carrot and parsnip on top. Put the onion on top of the carrot and parsnip, and the potato over all the other vegetables.

● Pour over the lamb stock, tuck in the rosemary, and cover the dish. Bake in the preheated oven for 1 hour.

● Increase the oven temperature to 200°C/400°F/Gas 6. Remove the cover, dot with butter, and cook for a further half-hour to brown the potatoes a little.

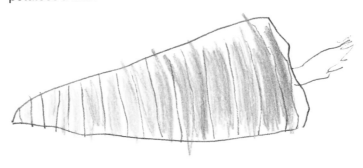

Lamb and apple pie

If you find it difficult to get your children to eat apples, try this recipe, making sure that you dice the apples small.

SERVES 4

For the pastry
450g (1lb) plain flour
115g (4oz) vegetable
    shortening, diced
115g (4oz) butter, diced
50ml (2fl oz) water

For the filling
450g (1lb) minced lamb
225g (8oz) carrots, peeled
    and diced
225g (8oz) onions, peeled
    and diced
225g (8oz) celery, diced
225g (8oz) apples, peeled,
    cored and diced
½ level teaspoon Marmite
25g (1oz) plain flour

The filling is suitable for freezing. Defrost and cook encased in pastry in the oven for 35–40 minutes as described in the recipe.

● Make the pastry as described on page 66 and leave to chill in the fridge for at least 30 minutes.

● In a frying pan dry-fry the minced lamb to brown it, then drain if necessary. Add the carrots, onions and celery to the mince, with just enough water to cover the meat – about 700ml (1¼ pints) – and simmer for 20–25 minutes, or until the onions and carrots are cooked.

● Add the apples and Marmite. Mix the flour with a little water, and pour through a sieve over the meat. Stir over heat for a further 10 minutes to thicken the sauce.

● Meanwhile preheat the oven to 190°C/375°F/Gas 5, and put in a baking sheet (a hot baking sheet helps make the base of the pastry crisp).

● Allow the pastry to come back to room temperature, then roll out thinly. Line a 25cm (10in) ovenproof dish with the majority of the pastry (leave enough for a lid). Add the meat mixture to the dish, and form a lid with the remaining pastry. Brush the edges of the pastry with water, cover the base and filling with the lid and pinch together. Brush the top and sides of the pastry with a little water (or with some beaten egg if you like).

● Put the dish on the hot baking sheet in the preheated oven and bake for 35–40 minutes until golden brown.

Spicy lamb burgers ▶

This recipe was devised at the new training kitchen in Essex, and I have to thank Simon Owens, who works with me there. Everyone who eats the burgers thinks they are great. Serve in a halved warm pitta bread or mini burger buns, with salad and a fresh mint and yoghurt dressing (see page 234), or a salad of chopped carrots, tomato and cucumber. Add a squeeze of lemon to the lamb burgers once they are cooked.

MAKES ABOUT 16

½ bunch fresh coriander (with stalks), chopped
175g (6oz) onions, peeled and finely chopped
1 small red chilli, deseeded and finely chopped
1 tablespoon olive oil
1kg (2¼ lb) minced lamb
1 teaspoon ground cumin
½ teaspoon ground turmeric
½ teaspoon ground coriander
1 egg, beaten

Suitable for freezing
before cooking.

● Wash the fresh coriander thoroughly.

● Cook the onion and chilli in the olive oil in a frying pan until golden and soft. Leave to cool a little.

● Combine all the ingredients in a large bowl and stir until thoroughly mixed. Divide the mixture into small burgers, shaping them as you wish; but it should make about 16.

● Place on a baking sheet and cook under a hot grill for 3–4 minutes on each side, or for 3–4 minutes on each side on the barbecue.

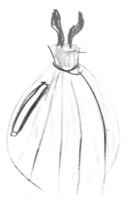

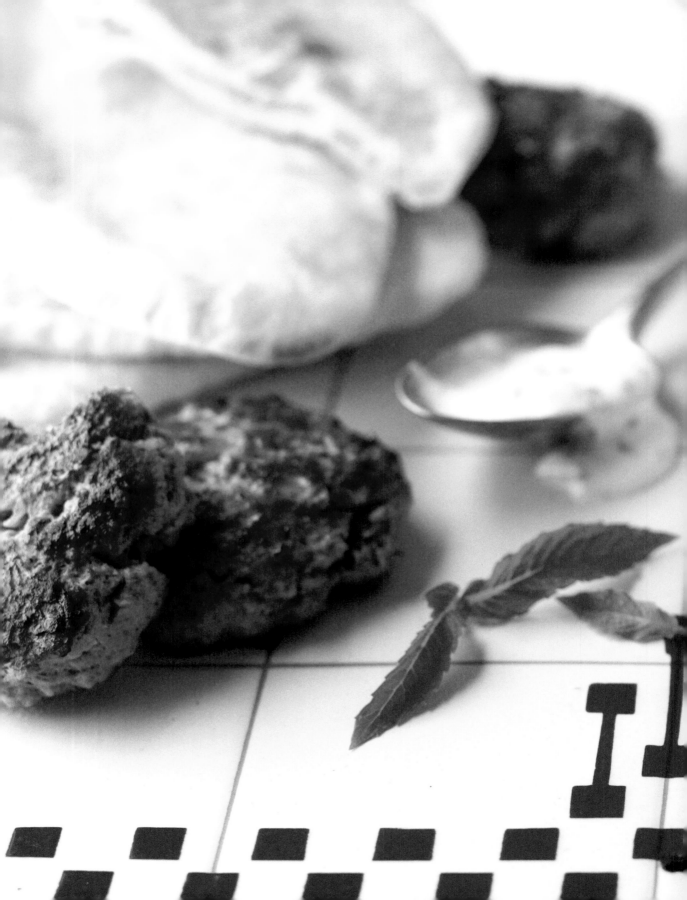

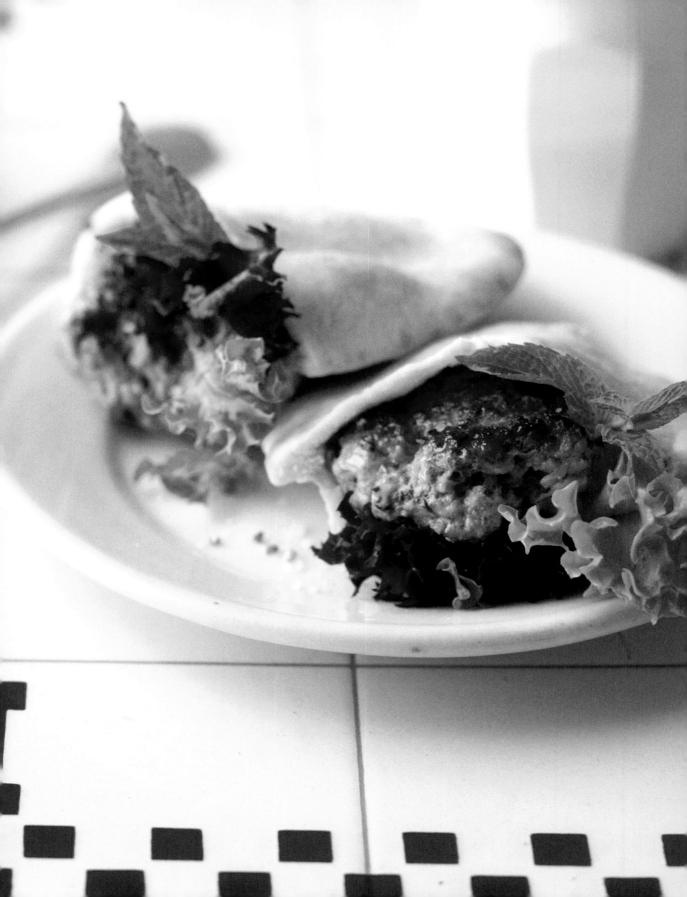

Steak and kidney pie

Sometimes children do not like offal. I have introduced kidney in this recipe, but I use lambs' because they are sweeter than pigs' and do not have such a strong flavour. Ask your butcher to remove the core from the kidney, as this is quite a fiddly job. The meat could be cooked the night before. If you do this, cool quickly and place covered in the fridge. Another tip: for a more sophisticated version, replace the water with Guinness, which is very good (just ask my husband!).

SERVES 4

For the pastry
225g (8oz) plain flour
55g (2oz) butter, diced
55g (2oz) vegetable shortening, diced
25ml (1fl oz) water
milk

For the filling
olive oil
900g (2lb) stewing steak, trimmed and finely diced
175g (6oz) onions, peeled and sliced
175g (6oz) lambs' kidneys, cored and finely diced
1 teaspoon Marmite
a few drops of Worcestershire sauce
450ml (16fl oz) water or beef stock (see page 223)
25g (1oz) plain flour

❄ The meat is suitable for freezing. Defrost, cover with pastry, and cook as in the recipe.

● Make the pastry as described on page 66. Leave to rest in the fridge for at least 30 minutes.

● Heat a little oil in a large pan, then add the stewing steak and seal on all sides. Remove from the pan and set aside. Cook the onions in the same pan for 5–10 minutes until soft and brown, adding a little more oil if necessary.

● Put the meat, onion and kidneys into a large saucepan. Mix the Marmite and Worcestershire sauce with the water or stock and pour it over the meat. Cover with a lid, and simmer for 45–60 minutes until the meat is tender. (Or cook in a preheated oven at 150°C/300°F/Gas 2 for 1¼ hours.)

● Mix the flour with a little water and pour through a sieve over the meat, stirring all the time. Continue to cook for 5–10 minutes until the sauce has thickened.

● When ready to cook the pie, remove the pastry from the fridge and bring it to room temperature. Preheat the oven to 200°C/400°F/Gas 6.

● Put the meat in a large pie dish. Roll out the pastry on a lightly floured surface and trim to about 5cm (2in) larger than your pie dish. Cut off a 2.5cm (1in) strip from all round the sheet and press this on to the rim of the pie dish. Brush the pastry with a little milk, then position the remaining pastry on top to form a lid. Press the edges together to seal then, using a sharp knife and your thumb, scallop the edges. Make a slit in the centre of the pastry to let the steam escape. Decorate the top with leaves cut from leftover pastry trimmings if you like. Brush all over the top of the pastry with a little milk.

● Bake in the preheated oven for 30–35 minutes until the pastry is golden brown.

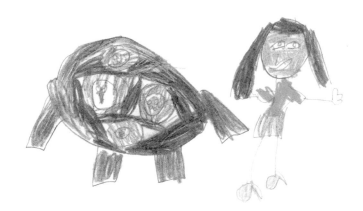

Braised brisket of beef with barley

This is delicious served with mashed potato and French beans or buttered spring cabbage. It's an ideal recipe for a slow-cooker (see page 70); the smell as you come into your house will be fantastic.

SERVES 4 (with leftovers)

1 x 900g (2lb) piece boned and rolled brisket of beef
25g (1oz) plain flour, seasoned with salt and pepper
2 tablespoons vegetable oil
115g (4oz) lean bacon rashers, rinded and chopped
450g (1lb) onions, peeled and diced
225g (8oz) carrots, peeled and diced
115g (4oz) celery, diced
1 tablespoon Marmite, dissolved in 700ml (1¼ pints)
    boiling water, or beef stock (see page 223)
55g (2oz) pearl barley

Freeze after cooking, then defrost and reheat in a moderate oven for about 30–35 minutes, adding extra stock if necessary.

● Roll the meat in the seasoned flour. Heat the oil in a large saucepan or casserole, then brown the meat on all sides. Set the meat aside.

● Add the bacon and vegetables to the oil in the pan, and fry until softened. Add the stock, season with salt and pepper, and put the meat on the bed of vegetables. Cover the pan and simmer on top of the stove for 45 minutes.

● Preheat the oven to 170°C/300°F/Gas 3.

● Add the barley to the casserole, stir and cover again, and place in the preheated oven for another 1½ hours. Turn the meat occasionally. If it looks as if it is drying up, add a bit more stock from time to time.

● Remove from the oven and leave to rest for about 10 minutes before carving.

Cottage pie

This dish used to be made with leftovers, but I make it with fresh butcher's mince. Hopefully once you've used this recipe, you'll realize how good it is.

SERVES 4

450g (1lb) minced beef
freshly ground black pepper
225g (8oz) onions, peeled and finely chopped
350g (12oz) carrots, peeled and diced
225g (8oz) swede, peeled and diced
1 sprig fresh rosemary
450g (1lb) potatoes, peeled and cut into 1cm (½in) slices
2 teaspoons Marmite
25g (1oz) plain flour
25g (1oz) butter, melted
85g (3oz) Cheddar cheese, grated

Suitable for freezing before adding the potato topping. Defrost, cover with potatoes, and reheat in a moderate oven, about 35 minutes, until piping hot.

● Preheat the oven to 200°C/400°F/Gas 6.

● In a large saucepan dry-fry the meat until it is brown, stirring. Grind over a little black pepper.

● Add the onion, carrot, swede and rosemary to the meat, with just enough water to cover – about 600ml (1 pint) – and simmer until the meat and vegetables are cooked, about 30–35 minutes.

● Meanwhile, place the potatoes in a pan of water, and par-boil for about 5 minutes. Drain.

● Add the Marmite to the meat, and cook for a further 10 minutes. Remove and discard the sprig of rosemary. Blend the flour with a little cold water, and add to the meat through a sieve, stirring carefully until the mixture thickens slightly.

● Pour the meat mixture into a casserole dish, and arrange the potato slices on top of the meat. Brush with the melted butter. Bake in the preheated oven until golden brown, about 30–35 minutes. About 5 minutes before the end of the cooking time, take the casserole out of the oven and sprinkle with the grated cheese. Return to the oven until the cheese has melted and become golden brown.

137

Boeuf bourguignon

Open up your child's taste-buds with this classic dish (minus the red wine). Serve it with mashed potato – or, even better, try mashed sweet potato.

SERVES 4

8 shallots
450g (1lb) lean stewing steak, diced
25g (1oz) plain flour
2 tablespoons olive oil
1 garlic clove, peeled and crushed
175g (6oz) bacon, rinded and diced
1 tablespoon Marmite, dissolved in 600ml (1 pint)
   boiling water, or beef stock (see page 223)
1 tablespoon tomato purée
1 bouquet garni (bay leaf, sprig of parsley, etc.)
175g (6oz) button mushrooms, wiped

❄

Freeze after cooking. Defrost and reheat thoroughly.

● Preheat the oven to 180°C/350°F/Gas 4.

● Put the unpeeled shallots in a small saucepan and cover with boiling water. Leave for a few minutes, then drain (this soaking makes them easier to peel). When cool enough to handle, remove the skins.

● Toss the beef in flour, and keep any remaining flour. Heat the olive oil in a frying pan, add half of the meat and brown on all sides to seal it. Remove with a slotted spoon and set aside, then repeat with the rest of the meat. Add the crushed garlic to the pan, stir well, then add the shallots and bacon and brown, about 5–10 minutes. Add the Marmite stock and the tomato purée, and stir well until the purée has dissolved. Add the bouquet garni.

● Transfer all the ingredients to a suitably sized ovenproof dish, cover and cook for approximately 1½ hours in the preheated oven.

● About 20 minutes before the end of cooking add the mushrooms. If necessary, thicken the juices with a little flour and water mixed together and strained into the dish through a sieve. Stir well, and return to the oven for the remaining 20 minutes.

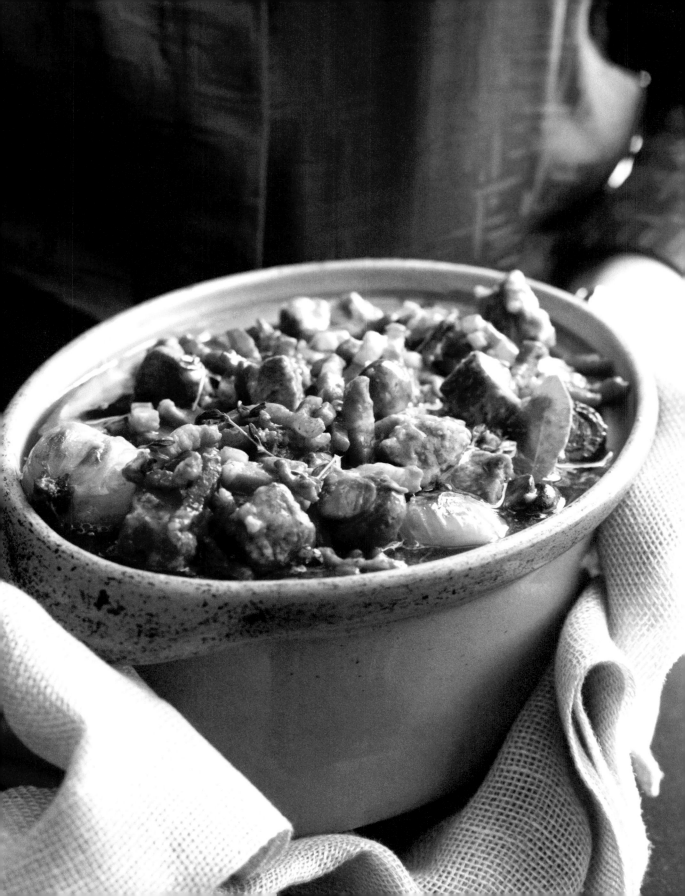

Cumberland pie

This is a twist on shepherd's or cottage pie, and I am sure your children will love it!

SERVES 4

900g (2lb) potatoes, peeled and quartered
50ml (2fl oz) milk, warmed
25g (1oz) butter
450g (1lb) good sausages, chopped into small pieces
olive oil
225g (8oz) onions, peeled and diced
1 garlic clove, peeled and crushed
225g (8oz) carrots, peeled and diced
4 peppers – 2 green and 2 red – deseeded and sliced
a pinch of dried thyme
2 x 400g cans chopped tomatoes

● Preheat the oven to 180°C/350°F/Gas 4.

● Place the potatoes in a saucepan, cover with water and bring to the boil. Simmer for about 15–20 minutes until soft, then drain and mash with the milk and butter. Leave in the saucepan.

● Meanwhile, put the sausage pieces in an ovenproof dish large enough to hold all the ingredients. Lightly brown the sausages in the preheated oven for 10 minutes.

● Heat a little olive oil in a pan, and cook the onions, garlic, carrots and peppers with the thyme until soft, about 8 minutes, then add the tomatoes and their juice. Stir the mixture and bring to the boil. Pour the mixture over the sausages in the casserole. Then spoon the mash on top, and fork it so that the potato covers the sausage mixture.

● Return the casserole to the oven and bake for 40 minutes.

Cheese, sausage and spinach pie

Spinach may look a lot when you buy it, but it soon cooks down, and it's a great way to get some iron into the kids. You could also call this dish 'Popeye Pie', which might appeal!

SERVES 4–6

For the cheese sauce
55g (2oz) butter
55g (2oz) plain flour
600ml (1 pint) milk
175g (6oz) Cheddar
    cheese, grated
1 teaspoon grain mustard
a pinch of freshly grated
    nutmeg

For the filling
450g (1lb) potatoes,
    peeled and quartered
15g (½oz) butter
olive oil
450g (1lb) good sausages,
    sliced into chunks
900g (2lb) fresh spinach
55g (2oz) Cheddar cheese, grated

● Preheat the oven to 190°C/375°F/Gas 5.

● To make the cheese sauce, melt the butter in a saucepan then add the flour and cook until sandy in texture. Add most of the milk (saving a little for the potatoes), whisking all the time, until the sauce thickens. Continue to cook over a low heat for 3–5 minutes. Add the cheese, grain mustard and nutmeg, and stir together. Put to one side.

● Place the potatoes in a saucepan, cover with water and bring to the boil. Simmer for about 15–20 minutes until soft, then drain and mash with the remaining milk and the butter. Leave in the saucepan.

● Heat a tablespoon of olive oil in a pan and cook the sausage slices until brown.

● Wash the spinach under cold running water, then place in a saucepan with just the water clinging to the leaves. Cook it for 5 minutes or until the leaves wilt, then strain. Get rid of the remaining water by very gently squeezing the spinach between two plates.

● Spread the spinach over the base of a large ovenproof dish, then add the sausage. Pour the cheese sauce over the top, and cover with the mashed potato. Sprinkle with the grated cheese, and cook in the preheated oven until golden brown, about 15–20 minutes.

Penne pasta with sausage in tomato sauce

A very good friend of mine tells me that she and her children often have penne pasta for tea as it is so quick to cook and good for you. Helen, you may like to try this, as the children have told me they get fed up with plain pasta and tomato sauce ...

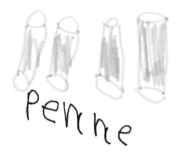

Penne

SERVES 4

4 large, good-quality Cumberland or other pork sausages
1 tablespoon olive oil
250g (9oz) penne pasta
about 55g (2oz) Parmesan cheese, freshly grated

For the tomato sauce
300ml (10fl oz) water
4 tablespoons tomato purée
250g (9oz) cherry tomatoes
2 tablespoons chopped fresh basil
1 garlic clove, peeled and crushed
1 teaspoon caster sugar
1 teaspoon white wine vinegar

● Fry the sausages in the olive oil until cooked through and brown, about 15–20 minutes. Drain on kitchen paper and when cool enough to handle cut into 1cm (½in) slices. Put to one side.

● For the sauce, pour the water into a pan, add the tomato purée and stir until dissolved. Add the cherry tomatoes, basil, garlic, sugar and vinegar, and bring to the boil. Cook until reduced by half, about 5–10 minutes.

● Meanwhile bring a pan of water to the boil and cook the pasta for about 5–10 minutes until soft. Drain and pour into a medium ovenproof dish.

● Preheat the grill.

● Arrange the sausage on top of the pasta, pour over the tomato sauce, and sprinkle with the Parmesan cheese. Grill for about 5 minutes to melt the cheese.

Bacon in the hole with onion gravy

This is a twist on the normal toad in the hole. It doesn't work as well in one big dish, so use smaller patty dishes – this quantity will make about 24. Adding vinegar to a batter mixture seems unusual, but it's a very Yorkshire thing to do!

SERVES 4–6

225g (8oz) plain flour
a pinch of black pepper
2 eggs
600–700ml (1–1¼ pints) milk
2 tablespoons malt vinegar
50ml (2fl oz) sunflower oil
275g (9½ oz) bacon,
   rinded and diced

For the onion gravy
55g (2oz) butter
2–3 onions, peeled and sliced
a pinch of caster sugar
1 tablespoon plain flour
200ml (7fl oz) stock
   (see page 223)
1 teaspoon Marmite
a dash of Worcestershire sauce

These little Yorkshire puddings freeze well once cooked and puffed up. Defrost and reheat in a moderate oven. The onion gravy freezes well too, ready for you to warm through at any time.

● Put the flour and the pepper into a large bowl. Make a well in the centre and add the eggs. Gradually whisk in 600ml (1 pint) of the milk, along with the malt vinegar. Beat well until smooth, then put to one side to rest.

● Meanwhile, make the onion gravy. Melt the butter in a frying pan, add the onion and cook over a low heat for about 10–15 minutes until soft and golden brown. Turn frequently to prevent burning. A pinch of sugar will help the onions brown more quickly. Add the flour and stir for 1 minute, then add the stock, Marmite and Worcestershire sauce. Bring the gravy to the boil, and simmer for 5 minutes or so.

● Preheat the oven to 220°C/425°F/Gas 7. Divide the oil between the patty tins and put the tins into the oven to heat.

● Cook the bacon in a frying pan until crisp, but do not brown. Remove the patty tins from the oven, and quickly add a little bacon, about a teaspoon, to each. Pour in the batter mixture almost to the top of each tin, and return to the oven. Do all this as quickly as you can. Bake until well-risen and golden brown, about 10–15 minutes. Serve with the hot onion gravy.

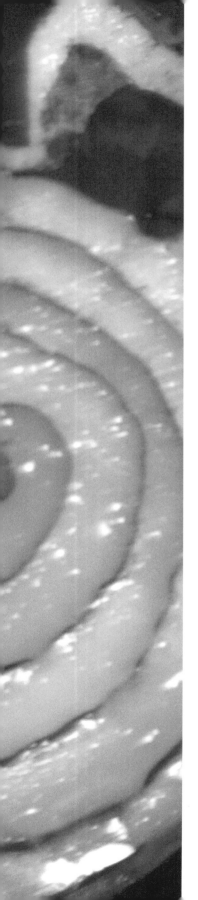

Bacon, bean and red pepper risotto

This one will hopefully really broaden children's taste-buds. It's quick and easy to make.

SERVES 4

350g (12oz) bacon, rinded and diced
olive oil
175g (6oz) red onions, peeled and sliced
3 celery sticks, sliced
1 red pepper, deseeded and thinly sliced lengthways
175g (6oz) brown rice
1 x 400g can haricot beans, drained and rinsed
1 litre (1¾ pints) vegetable stock (see page 223)
2 tablespoons grated Cheddar or Parmesan cheese (optional)
a handful of fresh basil leaves (optional)

● In a frying pan dry-fry the bacon until brown, about 3–4 minutes. Remove with a slotted spoon and put to one side. Warm a little olive oil in the same pan, and cook the onion, celery and pepper slices for 5–10 minutes until golden brown.

● Put the rice in a saucepan, add the vegetable stock and bring to the boil. Cover and simmer for 30–35 minutes until the rice is tender, stirring occasionally to prevent sticking.

● About 5 minutes before the rice is ready, stir in the beans, vegetables and bacon.

● If using, sprinkle the cheese and basil over each portion as you serve.

BBQ spare ribs

These are great served with the egg-fried rice on page 184, and are so easy to prepare. Kids enjoy eating with their hands, and they love these savoury tastes.

SERVES 4

1.1kg (2½lb) pork spare ribs

For the marinade
3 tablespoons tomato sauce
2 tablespoons Worcestershire sauce
2 tablespoons soft brown sugar
1 tablespoon soy sauce
½ teaspoon English mustard

● Mix all the marinade ingredients together in a large bowl. Place the spare ribs into a sealable plastic bag, and add the marinade. Rub the marinade into the ribs and chill in the fridge for at least 30–40 minutes (or overnight).

● Preheat the oven to 200°C/400°F/Gas 6.

● Place the ribs on a shallow baking tray, and bake in the preheated oven for 30–40 minutes until thoroughly cooked through and brown. Turn halfway through the cooking time.

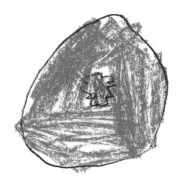

Honey-baked gammon

A piece of gammon is a practical joint for a family Sunday lunch. Most are sold vacuum packed with cooking instructions, but try your local butcher for the best quality and tastiest meat. Serve it with a parsley sauce (see page 61) and mashed potato and peas, or a vegetable mash (see page 201).

SERVES 4

450g (1lb) middle-cut boneless gammon
1 tablespoon English mustard
1 tablespoon runny honey

● Preheat the oven to 170°C/325°F/Gas 3.

● Soak the gammon according to the supplier's instructions.

● Wrap the gammon loosely in foil so that there is room for air to circulate. Place the parcel in a tin and cook for 20 minutes per 450g (1lb).

● Meanwhile, mix the mustard and honey together in a small bowl.

● About 10 minutes before the end of cooking, remove the gammon from the oven and open up the foil. Remove the skin, if there is any. Score the fat, in a diamond pattern if you like, then spoon the mustard and honey glaze all over it.

● Increase the heat of the oven to 220°C/425°F/Gas 7, and return the gammon to the oven for the last 10 minutes, basting from the tin if it looks at all dry.

● Once it is cooked, remove the gammon from the oven, wrap it back up in its foil and allow to stand for 15–20 minutes before carving and serving.

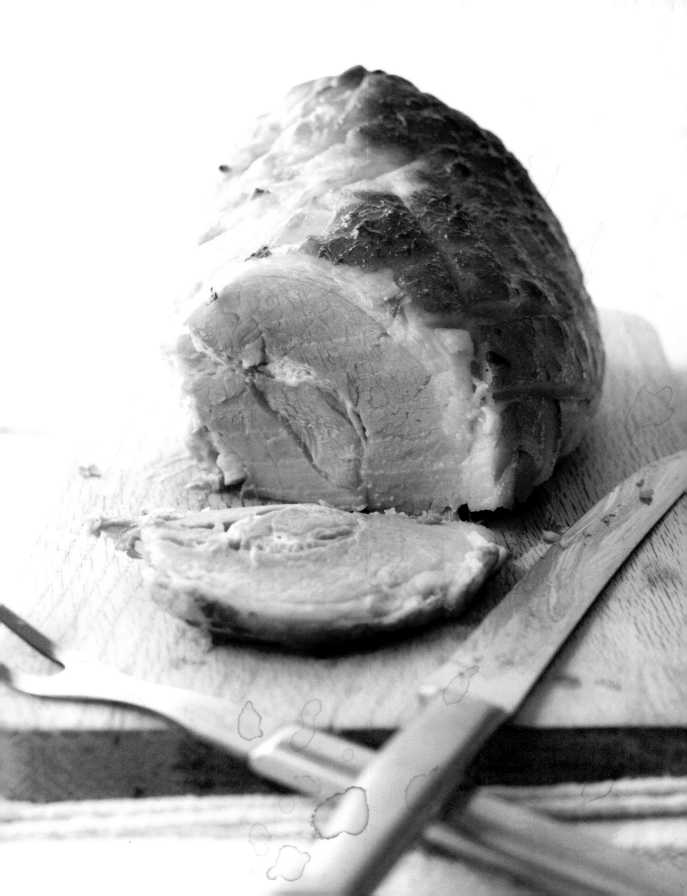

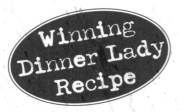

Winning Dinner Lady Recipe

Chicken keema

I have chosen this as the winner from all the recipes we received from dinner ladies the length and breadth of the country. Ann O'Sullivan, group kitchen supervisor at Greenbank Primary School in Rochdale, sent it to me, saying the following: 'Greenbank School has approximately 90 per cent uptake of children from an ethnic minority background. This dish has been produced with the assistance of the kitchen supervisor and various people involved at the school. The children and staff enjoy this dish being available on the menu.'

SERVES 4

2 tablespoons vegetable oil
450g (1lb) boneless chicken
    breasts, skinned and diced
1x 400g can chopped tomatoes

For the curry paste
seeds from 1 black
    cardamom pod
2 cloves
½ teaspoon coarsely
    ground black pepper

1 teaspoon garlic powder
1 teaspoon ground coriander
½ teaspoon ground ginger
¼ teaspoon powdered cinnamon
¼ teaspoon ground turmeric
½ teaspoon mild chilli powder
¼ teaspoon salt
½ teaspoon ground cumin
1 bay leaf

❄️
This can be frozen after cooking.

Ann O'Sullivan suggests 'For Keema Aloo, add 350g (12oz) potatoes, peeled and cut into small pieces. For Keema Matar, add 115g (4oz) peas.'

● Heat a heavy-based frying pan or casserole dish and add the oil. Quickly cook the chicken pieces on each side to seal the meat, 1–2 minutes. Remove and set aside in a warm place.

● Grind the cardamom seeds with the cloves using a pestle and mortar, or use a heavy bowl and the end of a rolling pin. Mix all the spices together, including the bay leaf, and then add them to the pan and cook, stirring, for 1 minute. Add the tomatoes and 300ml (10floz) water (and the potatoes, if making Aloo). Cover and simmer for 20–25 minutes.

● Return the chicken to the pan (with the peas, if making Matar), and cook for a further 5 minutes.

● Serve with natural bio-live yoghurt mixed with chopped fresh coriander, boiled basmati rice and warm naan bread.

Moroccan chicken with apricots

I have added this Moroccan tagine recipe to encourage children to try different tastes. Serve it with rice or, more traditionally, with the fast-cooking couscous you can find these days.

SERVES 4

½ teaspoon ground turmeric
½ teaspoon ground ginger
½ teaspoon paprika
½ teaspoon powdered cinnamon
2 tablespoons olive oil
1 red onion, peeled and diced
225g (8oz) carrots, peeled and diced
450g (1lb) boneless chicken breasts, skinned and diced
600ml (1 pint) chicken stock (see page 223)
1 tablespoon tomato purée
juice of 1 orange
1 x 400g can chickpeas, drained and rinsed
115g (4oz) dried apricots, chopped

Double up the spices

leave out, doesn't add anything except to make it all a bit chicken stewish

This can be frozen after cooking.

● Mix the spices together in a small bowl.

● Heat the olive oil in a large pan, add the spices, the onion and the carrot, and cook for about 5 minutes. Add the chicken and cook for 2–3 minutes, then add the stock, tomato purée, orange juice, chickpeas and apricots.

● Cook for a further 10 minutes, and serve.

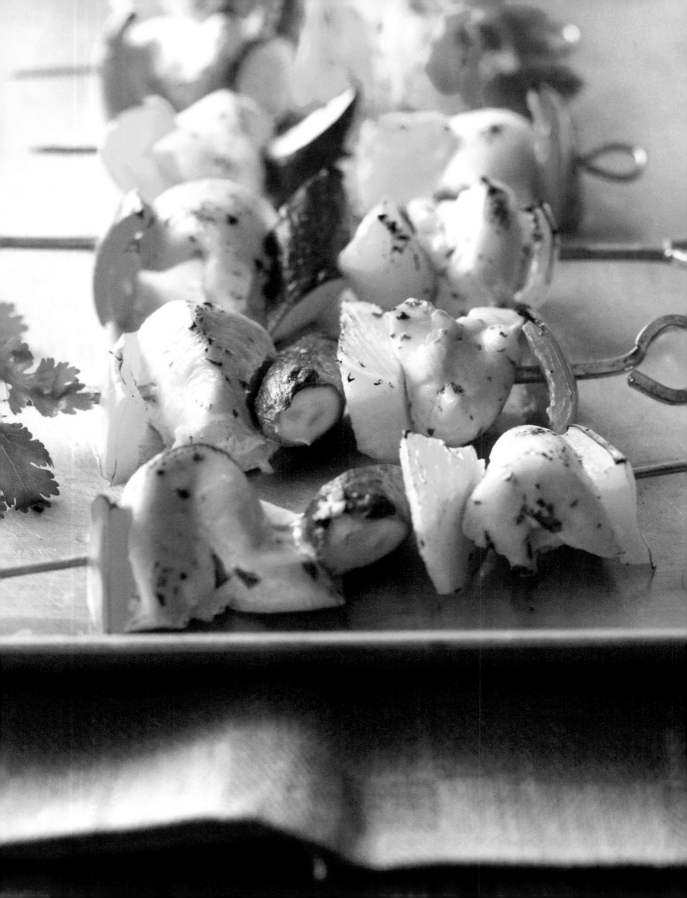

Chicken kebabs

You can vary the meat, using diced lamb or diced pork. You'll need eight skewers. If these are wooden, soak in cold water for at least an hour before using, which prevents them burning. You could assemble the kebabs the day before, but you must keep them in the fridge.

SERVES 4

350g (12oz) boneless chicken breasts, skinned and cut into
    2.5cm (1in) chunks
3 tablespoons runny honey
2 tablespoons natural bio-live yoghurt
1 tablespoon chopped fresh coriander
½ green pepper and ½ red pepper, deseeded
225g (8oz) fresh pineapple, peeled
115g (4oz) courgettes, trimmed

● Put the chicken in a bowl. In a separate bowl, mix together the honey, yoghurt and coriander. Pour over the diced chicken, stir well, cover and place in the fridge for half an hour (or longer).

● Preheat the grill. Cut all the fruit and vegetables into chunks the same size as the chicken.

● Thread pieces of the chicken, fruit and vegetables alternately on the skewers until they are full. Cover any exposed part of wooden skewers with foil. Place on a lightly oiled grill rack, and grill for about 10–15 minutes, turning, until the chicken is cooked through.

Chicken Maryland

This dish is like the 'fried chicken' that is so famous in America, and that we have become familiar with through a national chain of fast-food shops. A traditional chicken Maryland is deep-fried and served with corn fritters, rolls of bacon and fried banana. This recipe is baked in the oven so is much less fatty. You could serve the chicken and fritters with the pineapple and mango salsa on page 232.

SERVES 4

140g (5oz) fresh wholemeal breadcrumbs (or finely crushed Ritz or TUC biscuits)
1 teaspoon each of paprika and mustard powder
¼ teaspoon cayenne pepper
1½ teaspoons garlic granules
8 chicken thighs, skinned
115g (4oz) plain flour

2 eggs, beaten
1 tablespoon vegetable oil

For the corn fritters
1 x 340g can sweetcorn
115g (4oz) plain flour
1 egg
150ml (5fl oz) milk
a little vegetable oil

● To make the corn fritters, drain the sweetcorn, and put it in the food processor with the flour, egg and milk. Blend until smooth. Leave for 30 minutes before cooking.

● Preheat the oven to 200°C/400°F/Gas 6.

● Mix the breadcrumbs or crushed biscuits with the spices. Roll the chicken thighs in the flour, then dip into the beaten egg, and then into the spiced crumbs. Shake off any loose crumbs.

● Oil a baking sheet, lay the coated thighs on it and bake in the preheated oven for 20 minutes. Turn over and bake for another 20 minutes.

● Meanwhile, cook the corn fritters. Heat a little oil in a frying pan, and add tablespoons of the corn batter. Fry until golden, about 2–3 minutes on each side.

● Serve the chicken hot with the corn fritters, and a salad on the side.

Chicken tikka

For a genuine chicken tikka, a tandoor oven is required. We shall have to make do with the grill, turned up to its highest heat (or you could bake the chicken pieces, without skewers, in the oven instead). Serve with a small salad, and some naan or pitta bread, or as part of a main-course meal, with rice and a vegetable curry (see page 181). The skewers are good dipped into some mango chutney. A friend of mine, Kemi, told me her children love this recipe. If you are using wooden skewers, soak them in water first to prevent them burning.

SERVES 4

4 boneless chicken breasts, skinned and cut into 2.5cm (1in) pieces
2 tablespoons lemon juice
140g (5oz) natural bio-live yoghurt
1 large garlic clove, peeled and crushed
1 tablespoon chopped fresh coriander (optional)
1 x 2.5cm (1in) piece fresh root ginger, grated
a few chilli flakes (optional)
1 teaspoon garam masala
½ teaspoon ground coriander

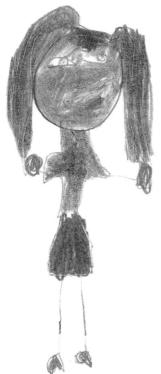

● Put the chicken pieces in a dish and sprinkle with the lemon juice.

● Mix the yoghurt with the garlic, coriander (if using) and spices, and pour over the chicken. Leave to marinate for at least 2 hours in the fridge. (This could be done the night before, if serving for a lunch at the weekend.)

● Preheat the grill to its highest temperature.

● Brush off and discard the marinade, and thread the chicken pieces towards one end of thin wooden or metal skewers. If using wooden skewers, cover any exposed wood to prevent burning. Grill until tender, turning the skewers, for about 8–10 minutes.

Chicken and prawn paella

You could use chicken wings for this recipe, but boneless chicken is safer for little ones. The children at St Peter's often used to ask me to make paella, but unfortunately I didn't have a large enough pan!

SERVES 4

2 tablespoons olive oil
1 garlic clove, peeled and finely chopped
450g (1lb) boneless chicken breasts, skinned and cut into strips
1 red pepper, deseeded and cut into thin strips
3 spring onions, sliced
500ml (18fl oz) chicken stock (see page 223)
250g (9oz) brown rice
175g (6oz) uncooked tiger prawns
8 cherry tomatoes, halved
100g (3½ oz) frozen peas
2 tablespoons chopped fresh parsley
juice of 1 lemon
freshly ground black pepper

● Heat the olive oil in a large frying pan. Cook the garlic gently until golden, then add half the chicken and cook until brown and tender, about 5 minutes. Remove from the pan and put to one side. Cook the remaining chicken in the same way, and remove from the pan. Cook the pepper strips and spring onions in the same pan for about 1–2 minutes. Remove and set aside.

● Add the stock and rice to the pan and cook, stirring occasionally, over a moderate heat for 20–25 minutes until the rice is cooked. Return the cooked peppers, spring onion and chicken to the pan and add the prawns, cherry tomatoes and peas. Continue to cook for a further 5 minutes.

● Take off the heat and leave to stand for 5 minutes before serving. Mix in the parsley, lemon juice and pepper as you serve.

Sesame chicken nuggets

This is a twist on the real chicken nugget recipe I gave in my last book, as I am trying to get the children to eat seeds now. And of course they can help you with this recipe as well.

SERVES 4

225g (8oz) sesame seeds
¼ teaspoon garlic powder
¼ teaspoon paprika
1 egg, beaten
125ml (4fl oz) milk
900g (2lb) boneless chicken breasts, skinned and cut into
    5cm (2 in) pieces
olive oil

● Preheat the oven to 200°C/400°F/Gas 6.

● Put the sesame seeds, garlic powder and paprika in a bowl, and mix well. Scatter over a large baking tray.

● Beat the egg in a large bowl with the milk, then add the chicken pieces in batches. Transfer the chicken pieces to the baking tray and coat them well in the flavoured seeds.

● Arrange the chicken pieces on a lightly oiled baking tray and bake in the preheated oven for 10 minutes until brown, crisp and cooked through.

Oriental chicken stir-fry

Stir-frying is a quick and easy way to prepare a great healthy meal after a hard day's work. There are a few ideas here.

SERVES 4

2 tablespoons soy sauce
juice of 1 large orange
450g (1lb) boneless chicken breasts, skinned and cut into strips
2 tablespoons olive oil
1 garlic clove, peeled and finely chopped
1 x 1cm (½ in) piece fresh root ginger, peeled and grated (optional)
1 green or red pepper, deseeded and cut into thin strips
6 spring onions, roughly chopped
2 teaspoons cornflour
300ml (10fl oz) chicken stock (see page 223)

● Combine the soy sauce and orange juice in a large bowl. Add the chicken strips and mix well. Cover with clingfilm and chill for about 1 hour.

● Heat the olive oil in a frying pan, and brown the chicken, in two batches, for about 5 minutes. Remove with a slotted spoon and put aside. Add the garlic and ginger (if using) to the oil left in the pan and cook over a moderate heat for 1–2 minutes. Add the peppers and spring onions, and cook for 5–6 minutes.

● Mix the cornflour with a little of the chicken stock. Return the chicken to the pan with the cornflour-stock mix and the remaining chicken stock. Continue to cook for a further 5 minutes until the chicken is thoroughly cooked.

Variations
● Try thin strips of beef – preferably a tender cut like fillet or rump – instead of chicken. Omit the orange juice and chicken stock and use beef stock instead. Or simply use thin strips of pork instead of the chicken.

● Use raw peeled tiger prawns instead of chicken, and stir-fry for 1 minute. Add 1 tablespoon lemon juice and the finely grated rind of 1 lemon. Use fish stock instead of chicken stock and lime juice instead of orange juice.

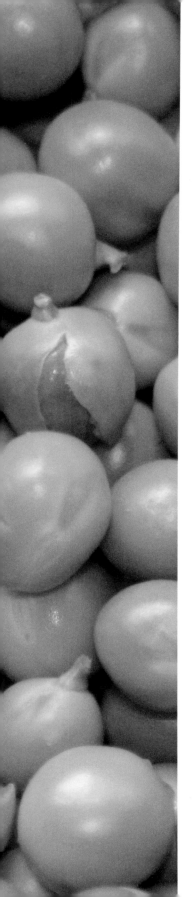

Chicken and vegetable risotto

Try sprinkling 115g (4oz) grated Cheddar cheese over the risotto when it is cooked. Cover with a lid, and leave for a few minutes until the cheese has melted. Serve immediately.

SERVES 4

450g (1lb) boneless chicken breasts, skinned and cut into strips
2 tablespoons olive oil
115g (4oz) onions, peeled and diced
115g (4oz) carrots, peeled and diced
1 garlic clove, peeled and crushed
225g (8oz) risotto rice
600ml (1 pint) boiling chicken stock (see page 223)
85g (3oz) frozen peas
85g (3oz) frozen sweetcorn

● Fry the chicken in half the olive oil for about 5–6 minutes, then remove to a bowl. Add the remaining oil to the pan, and fry the onion, carrot and garlic until soft, about another 5–6 minutes. Add the rice and stir so that each grain is covered in the oil and vegetables.

● Add the hot stock to the rice. Simmer, covered, until the liquid has been absorbed, about 15–20 minutes. Stir every now and then.

● Add the chicken, peas and sweetcorn, and cook for a further 5–10 minutes. This dish should be moist but not sloppy.

Chicken, pasta and sweetcorn medley

This would make a delicious dish for vegetarians – if you omitted the chicken, of course!

SERVES 4

175g (6oz) wholemeal spaghetti
300g (10½ oz) boneless chicken breasts, skinned and diced
olive oil
300g (10½ oz) spring onions
85g (3oz) frozen peas
85g (3oz) frozen sweetcorn

For the cheese sauce
25g (1oz) butter
25g (1oz) plain flour
600ml (1 pint) milk
115g (4oz) Cheddar cheese, grated
a pinch of cayenne pepper

● In a large saucepan of boiling water cook the spaghetti until al dente (just cooked, not too soft), about 10 minutes. Drain well and keep warm.

● Meanwhile, stir-fry the diced chicken in a little olive oil for 5–10 minutes. Remove with a slotted spoon and set to one side in a deep ovenproof dish, along with the cooked spaghetti. Cut the green part of the spring onion into 5mm (¼in) lengths and finely slice the white parts. Stir-fry the spring onions, peas and sweetcorn in a little olive oil for 2–3 minutes. Add to the chicken.

● To make the sauce, melt the butter in a pan, add the flour and cook until sandy in colour and texture. Add the milk, whisking all the time, and when the sauce is smooth and has thickened add the cheese, keeping a little back for the topping. Stir in the cayenne.

● Preheat the grill.

● Pour the cheese sauce over the chicken and spaghetti, and sprinkle with the remaining cheese. Put under the preheated grill and cook until sizzling and golden on top, about 5 minutes. Serve immediately.

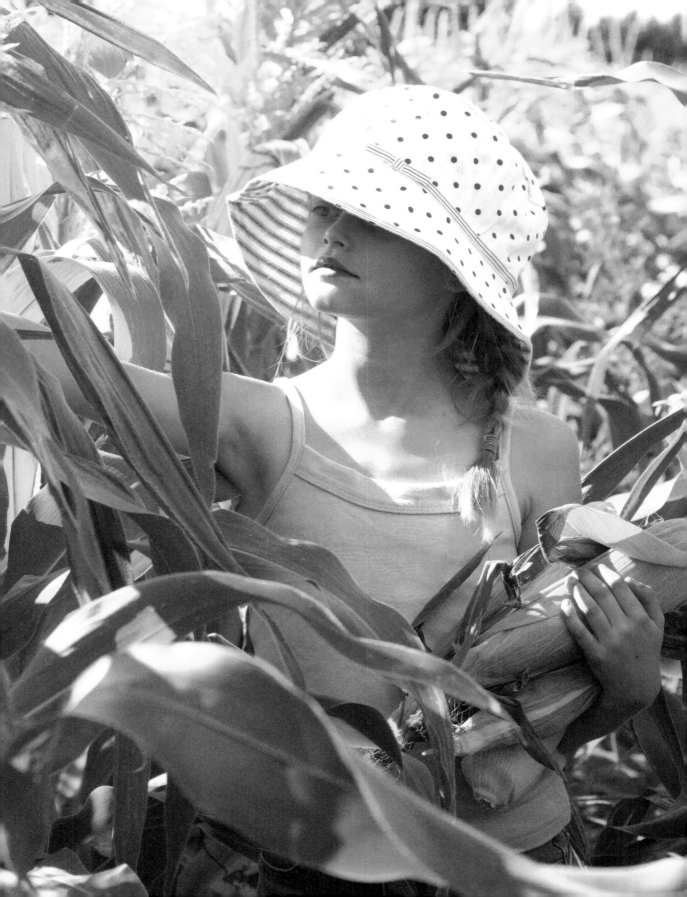

Fish and no chips...

Tuna with pasta twists

This dish combines three children's food favourites: pasta, tuna and a tomato sauce.

SERVES 4

3 tablespoons olive oil
1 onion, peeled and roughly chopped
1 garlic clove, peeled and crushed
2 beef tomatoes, cores removed and flesh roughly chopped
1 teaspoon mixed dried herbs (herbes de Provence)
1 teaspoon caster sugar
350g (12oz) fresh tuna steaks, or 1 x 200g can tuna in spring water
a little black pepper
225g (8oz) pasta twirls
grated Parmesan or Cheddar cheese to serve (optional)

● Heat 2 tablespoons of the olive oil in a frying pan and cook the onion and garlic for 3–4 minutes or until softened. Add the chopped tomato, mixed herbs, sugar and 200ml (7fl oz) water. Bring to the boil and simmer uncovered for 10–15 minutes.

● Meanwhile, heat the remaining oil in a heavy-based frying pan. If using fresh tuna, season with a little black pepper, and fry for 2 minutes on each side, or until just cooked. Set aside until cool enough to handle. Break the tuna into flakes, and add to the tomato sauce. If using canned tuna, drain well, flake and add to the tomato sauce.

● Cook the pasta in a large pan of boiling water according to the packet instructions. Drain, then stir into the tomato sauce. Serve with grated cheese (although it is not traditional with fish pasta in Italy).

fiorelli

I love pasta

Smoked haddock pancakes

These are really delicious, and of course fish is so good for all the family. You can use cod or salmon instead of smoked haddock. Choose haddock that is beige-gold, not bright yellow (which is dyed). This haddock sauce is good in pastry cases too. You can also add a couple of chopped hard-boiled eggs to the sauce, for extra protein.

SERVES 4

675g (1½lb) smoked haddock
300ml (10fl oz) milk
25g (1oz) butter
25g (1oz) plain flour
1 teaspoon Dijon mustard
140g (5oz) Cheddar cheese, grated
1 tablespoon chopped fresh parsley

For the pancakes
115g (4oz) plain flour
2 eggs, beaten
300ml (10fl oz) milk
sunflower oil for frying

The pancakes alone can be frozen; interleave them with foil, and wrap well.

● Preheat the oven to 180°C/350°F/Gas 4.

● Make the pancake batter first, so that it has time to stand and rest. Put the flour into a bowl and make a well in the centre. Add the eggs to the well, along with the milk, and whisk together for 3–4 minutes until all the flour is incorporated and there is plenty of air in the mixture.

● To poach the fish, put it with the milk in a pan, and bring up to the boil. Remove immediately from the heat, and leave to stand for 5 minutes. Strain the haddock, saving the milk for the sauce; you'll need 300ml (10fl oz), so make up with extra if necessary.

● For the sauce, melt the butter in a small saucepan, add the flour and cook over a low heat until sandy in texture, about 3–4 minutes. Gradually add the fishy milk, stirring constantly, and cook for a further 5–6 minutes until thickened. Remove from the heat, and stir in the mustard and cheese.

● Break the fish into rough chunks and add to the sauce, along with the parsley, mixing carefully so as not to break the fish into smaller pieces.

● To make the pancakes, heat about a tablespoon of the oil in a hot 25cm (10in) frying pan, swirl it around, and tip out into a metal or china jug. Pour in just enough batter to thinly coat the base of the pan. Cook over a moderately high heat for about 1 minute until golden brown. Turn or toss and cook the other side for 30–60 seconds until golden. Put to one side. Repeat with the remaining batter, using a little oil each time, and stacking the cooked pancakes on top of one another. You should make eight pancakes.

● Put about 2 tablespoons of the fish mixture in the centre of each of the pancakes. Roll up and place in a lightly oiled ovenproof dish. Cover the dish with foil and warm through in the preheated oven for about 15–20 minutes.

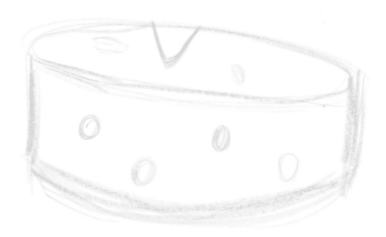

Crispy tuna and cheese nuggets

A little twist on fishcakes that children will like. Try to get tuna in spring water rather than in brine or oil. Serve the nuggets with home-made tomato ketchup and fat oven-baked potato chips.

SERVES 4

450g (1lb) potatoes, peeled and quartered
2 x 200g cans tuna in spring water, drained
225g (8oz) Cheddar cheese, grated
juice of 1 lemon
olive oil

For the coating
1 large egg
2 tablespoons milk
225g (8oz) fresh wholemeal breadcrumbs

● Boil the potatoes in water for 15–20 minutes until just soft, then mash (or push through a potato ricer, which makes a lump-free mash instantly). Put into a mixing bowl. Drain and flake the tuna, and add to the potato along with the cheese and lemon juice. Mix well and leave to rest in the fridge for about 30 minutes.

● Preheat the oven to 200°C/400°F/Gas 6.

● For the coating, whisk the egg and milk together. Place the breadcrumbs on a baking tray. Take the tuna mixture out of the fridge and roll into balls – wet hands are good. Dunk each ball in the egg mixture and then roll in breadcrumbs. Place on a lightly oiled baking sheet and repeat this until you have used all the mixture.

● Bake in the preheated oven until golden brown, about 15–20 minutes.

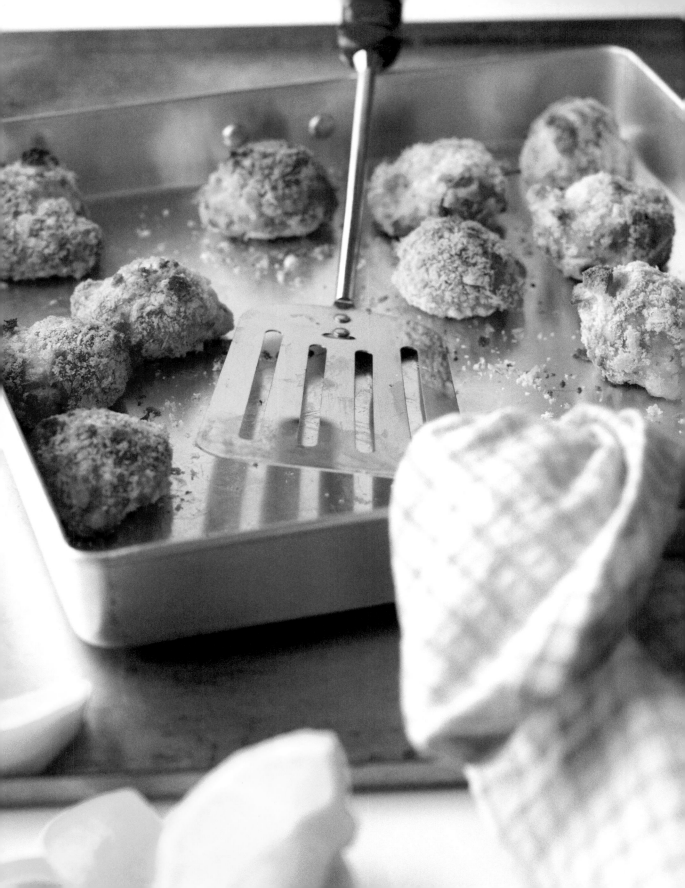

Fish and potato bake

This is one of my boys' favourites.

SERVES 4

450g (1lb) white fish (cod, coley, monkfish, or a mixture of all three)
700ml (1¼ pints) milk
450g (1lb) potatoes, peeled and quartered
55g (2oz) butter
115g (4oz) onions, peeled and finely diced
olive oil
175g (6oz) cherry tomatoes, washed and halved
25g (1oz) plain flour
1 teaspoon Dijon mustard
175g (6oz) Cheddar cheese, grated
2 tablespoons chopped fresh parsley
115g (4oz) brown breadcrumbs

Freeze once it has been assembled and before it is finally cooked.

● Preheat the oven to 180°C/ 350°F/Gas 4.

● Wash the fish thoroughly and dry on paper towels. Remove the skin (or you could ask your fishmonger to do this). Poach the fish in the milk for about 8–10 minutes. Remove from the milk with a slotted spoon, and place in a large ovenproof dish. Reserve the milk for later.

● Put the potatoes in a pan with water to cover and cook for 15–20 minutes until just soft. Drain and mash with 15g (½oz) of the butter and 90ml (3fl oz) of the reserved milk. Leave to one side.

● Fry the onion in a little olive oil until soft, about 5 minutes, then add to the fish. Dot the halved cherry tomatoes around the dish.

● Melt 25g (1oz) of the butter in a small pan, add the flour and cook until sandy in texture, about 2–3 minutes. Gradually add the remaining fishy milk, stirring all the time, and cook until smooth, about 3–4 minutes. Add the mustard, cheese and parsley.

● Pour the cheese sauce over the fish mixture, and mix gently. Place the mashed potato on the top and gently fork the potato so that it covers the fish. Sprinkle the breadcrumbs over the potato, and dot with the remaining butter. Bake in the preheated oven for 20–25 minutes until golden brown and piping hot.

Tuna fishcakes

This is ever-popular at St Peter's. Use salmon as well.

SERVES 4

500g (18oz) potatoes, peeled and quartered
25g (1oz) butter
6 spring onions, washed and finely chopped
2 heaped teaspoons English mustard
2 tablespoons finely chopped fresh parsley
1 tablespoon plain flour, plus extra for dusting
1 large egg yolk
1 x 200g can tuna in spring water, drained
3–4 tablespoons olive oil

Open freeze on a baking tray and then pack into freezer bags.

● Put the potatoes in a large saucepan, cover with water, bring to the boil and simmer until soft, about 15–20 minutes. Mash the potatoes, adding half the butter. Transfer to a large mixing bowl.

● Fry the spring onions for 1–2 minutes in the remaining butter to soften them. Add to the potatoes along with the mustard, chopped parsley and the flour. Mix well, then add the egg yolk and drained tuna, and mix well again.

● On a lightly floured surface, with floured hands, shape the mixture into eight rounds. Flatten lightly and dust with flour. Heat the olive oil in a large frying pan and fry the fishcakes gently for 5–6 minutes on each side until light gold in colour.

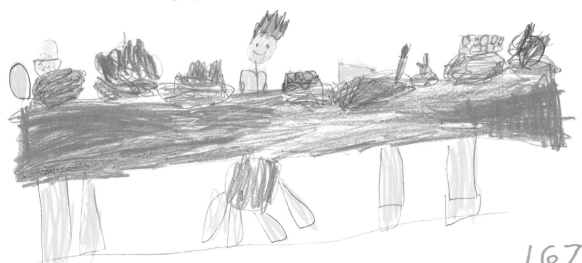

167

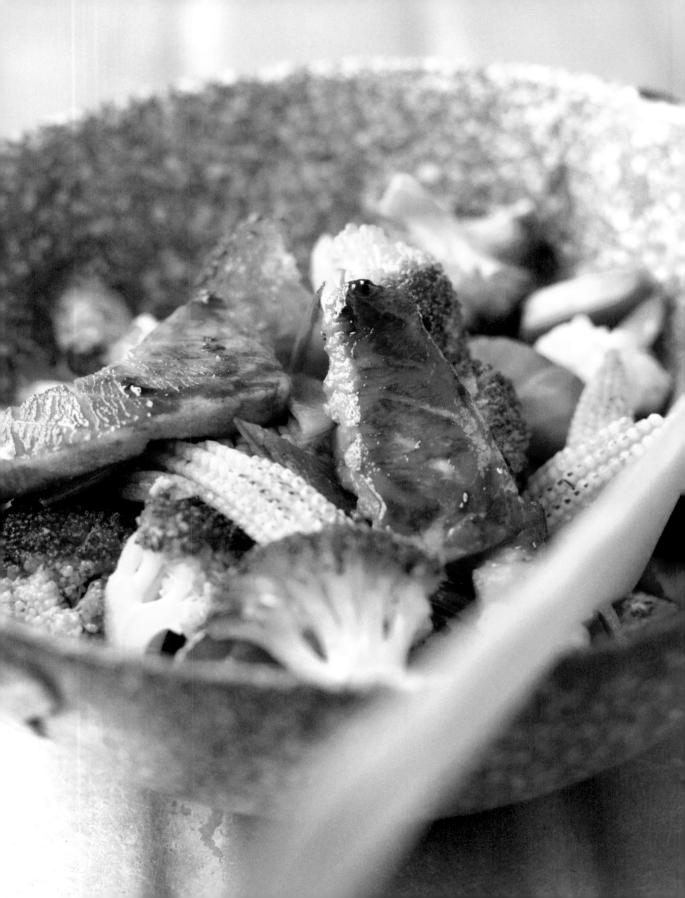

Oriental salmon and vegetable stir-fry

This is quick and easy, and the children can help you cook. It's a recipe that makes salmon go a long way. Serve with the egg-fried rice on page 184 or, better still, with thick rice noodles (follow the instructions on the packet). They could eat with chopsticks if they dare!

SERVES 4

115g (4oz) broccoli, cut into small florets
115g (4oz) cauliflower, cut into small florets
55g (2oz) baby sweetcorn
55g (2oz) mangetout
2 tablespoons soy sauce
2 tablespoons water
15g (½oz) brown sugar
1 tablespoon sunflower or vegetable oil
450g (1lb) skinless salmon fillets, cut into strips 1cm (½in) thick

● Prepare all the vegetables as appropriate. Make sure the broccoli and cauliflower are cut into small florets so that they cook quickly.

● Mix the soy sauce, water and sugar in a bowl, and put to one side.

● In a large frying pan or wok, heat the oil over a high heat. Add the broccoli and cauliflower and stir-fry, keeping them moving around the pan all the time. Add the sweetcorn and mangetout and cook for 4–5 minutes.

● Add the thin strips of salmon with the soy sauce mixture and stir-fry for 4–5 minutes until piping hot. Serve straight away.

Haddock lasagne

Lasagne doesn't always have to be a meat dish. Try this one for a change. Buy skinless haddock, or ask your fishmonger to skin the fillets for you. This is a great way to get children to eat vegetables too.

SERVES 4

olive oil
450g (1lb) skinned haddock fillets
150ml (5fl oz) milk
175g (6oz) onions, peeled
   and diced
1 celery stick, diced
175g (6oz) courgettes,
   washed and thinly sliced
175g (6oz) leeks, washed
   and thinly sliced
1 x 400g can chopped tomatoes

115g (4oz) frozen peas
a handful of fresh basil leaves
140g (5oz) pre-cooked lasagne

For the cheese sauce
25g (1oz) butter
25g (1oz) plain flour
600ml (1 pint) milk
1 teaspoon Dijon mustard
115g (4oz) Cheddar or Parmesan
   cheese, finely grated

Freeze once it has been assembled. Defrost thoroughly before finally cooking in the same temperature oven.

● Preheat the oven to 200°C/400°F/Gas 6, and grease the base of a suitable ovenproof dish.

● Wash the fish and pat dry on kitchen paper. Place the fish in a pan with enough milk to cover, and gently poach for 5–6 minutes. Put to one side, keeping the liquid.

● Heat a little olive oil in a saucepan and sauté the onion, celery, courgette and leek for about 5 minutes. Add the tomatoes and their juices, and the peas, and cook for 10 minutes. Add the basil at the last minute.

● To make the sauce, melt the butter in a small pan, then add the flour, and cook until the texture and colour are sandy. Add the milk and the reserved fishy milk, along with the mustard. Stir continuously until thickened and smooth, about 5 minutes. Stir in most of the cheese until melted.

● Arrange half the lasagne on the base of the dish, and cover with half of the vegetable sauce. Break the fish into pieces (removing any bones) and put these over the vegetables then pour over about half of the cheese sauce. Top with the remaining lasagne, vegetables and fish, and pour over the remaining sauce. Sprinkle with the rest of the grated cheese. Bake in the preheated oven until golden brown and the lasagne is soft, about 25–30 minutes.

Marinated fish parcels

You can use a variety of white fish, and salmon or fresh tuna in the summer, when you could cook on the barbecue. You will need four pieces of foil big enough to make airtight parcels.

SERVES 4

4 fish fillets, about 115–175g (4–6oz) each
2 tablespoons olive oil
1 tablespoon lemon juice
½ teaspoon mixed fresh herbs
½ teaspoon garlic powder
½ teaspoon rock salt
½ teaspoon black pepper

● Wash the fish under cold running water, and pat dry with kitchen paper. Place in a dish in one layer. Combine the olive oil, lemon juice and other ingredients in a bowl to make the marinade. Pour over the fish and place in the fridge for 2 hours, basting with the marinade once.

● Preheat the oven to 220°C/425°F/Gas 7.

● Remove the fish from the marinade, and place each fillet on a piece of foil. Spoon over the marinade, and fold the sides of the foil over to make a parcel. Place on a baking tray and bake in the preheated oven for 15–20 minutes.

Real fish fingers

These are almost as simple as the chicken nuggets in my last book. I have flavoured the breadcrumbs here with garlic salt, but you could add 2 tablespoons freshly grated Parmesan instead. Ask your fishmonger to skin the fish for you, or you can do it yourself. I serve the fingers with a salsa (see page 230–32) or tomato sauce, but wedges of baked potato are good too, as are boiled or steamed vegetables.

SERVES 4

85g (3oz) brown bread, sliced and toasted light brown
85g (3oz) white bread, sliced and toasted light brown
1 teaspoon garlic salt
1 egg
450g (1lb) fresh cod, haddock or salmon, skinned and sliced into
    2cm (¾in) strips

Freeze once breadcrumbed, and cook under the grill from frozen.

● Break the toast into pieces, crusts and all, and reduce to fine crumbs in the food processor. Place the breadcrumbs in a large deep tray, and mix with the garlic salt. Beat the egg in a large bowl.

● Dip a few strips of fish at a time in the egg, then transfer to the tray of breadcrumbs, coating thoroughly. Chill the fish fingers for 10 minutes (or longer).

● Preheat the grill.

● Arrange the fish fingers on a lightly greased wire rack in a grill tray to prevent the breadcrumbs going soggy. Grill for 8–10 minutes, turning, until the breadcrumbs have become brown and crisp.

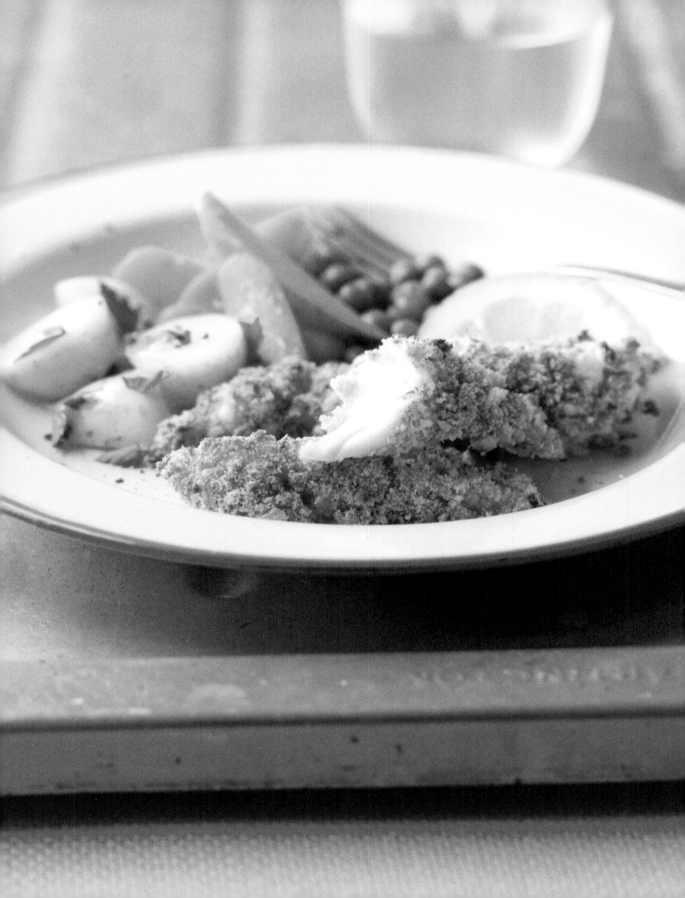

Fish stew

Trying to broaden children's palates can prove very wearing, so the younger you start the better. But if they don't like something, don't worry, go back and try again a few months later. Perseverance is the key. This delicious fish stew should appeal to them, and you can prepare the tomato base at least a day in advance.

SERVES 4

1kg (2¼lb) mixed white fish fillets
2 tablespoons olive oil
225g (8oz) onions, peeled and sliced
1 garlic clove, peeled and crushed
1 teaspoon dried thyme (or oregano)
225g (8oz) red peppers, deseeded and cut into small chunks
450g (1lb) soft and ripe plum tomatoes, halved
250ml (9fl oz) each of tomato passata and water
2 tablespoons chopped fresh parsley

● Rinse the fish and pat it dry on kitchen paper. Cut the fish into 2.5cm (1in) chunks and set aside.

● Heat the olive oil in a large saucepan and cook the onion, garlic and thyme for 5 minutes over a moderate heat. Do not brown. Add the pepper chunks and tomatoes, and continue to cook for about 5–10 minutes until the tomatoes are cooked down. Add the passata and water, and continue to simmer for another 10–15 minutes.

● Add the parsley and the fish, cover the pan and bring to the boil. Simmer for about 5 minutes, until the fish is tender. Serve in bowls with crusty bread to mop up the juices.

Cheesy fish

Children love sweetcorn and cherry tomatoes, but the Parmesan here adds a different and interesting flavour.

SERVES 4

4 pieces white fish fillet, about 115–175g (4–6oz) each
olive oil
115g (4oz) baby sweetcorn, cut into small pieces on the diagonal
115g (4oz) courgettes, trimmed and sliced
115g (4oz) cherry tomatoes, halved
8 basil leaves, torn
55g (2oz) fresh breadcrumbs
55g (2oz) Parmesan cheese, freshly grated

● Preheat the oven to 180°C/350°F/Gas 4.

● Rinse the fish and pat it dry on kitchen paper. Arrange in a lightly oiled ovenproof dish in one layer.

● Heat 1 tablespoon olive oil in a pan, and stir-fry the baby sweetcorn and courgette slices for 3–4 minutes. Scatter the vegetable mixture, along with the halved cherry tomatoes, across the fish in the dish. Top with the basil. Mix the breadcrumbs with the grated Parmesan and sprinkle over the vegetables and fish.

● Bake in the preheated oven for 15 minutes until the fish is cooked through, the vegetables are tender, and the breadcrumbs and cheese are crisp and golden on top.

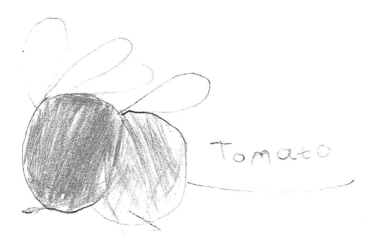

Tomato

175

For vegetarians

Vegetable burgers

I hope even meat-eaters will try this recipe, as it makes a change. Serve with the cucumber and yoghurt dip or the mango salsa on pages 234 and 230, and maybe jacket wedges.

SERVES 4

115g (4oz) carrots, peeled and cut in half
115g (4oz) potatoes, peeled and cut into large chunks
55g (2oz) sweet potato, peeled and cut into large chunks
115g (4oz) red onions, peeled and finely diced
3 tablespoons olive oil
55g (2oz) frozen sweetcorn
55g (2oz) wholemeal breadcrumbs
2 tablespoons chopped fresh herbs (basil and parsley)
2 eggs, beaten
2 tablespoons tomato purée
2 tablespoons natural bio-live yoghurt

Open freeze once shaped.

● Cook the carrot and potato in boiling water until tender, about 20 minutes. Add the sweet potato after 10 minutes. Drain, and mash the three vegetables together. Place in a bowl.

● Meanwhile, fry the onion in 1 tablespoon of the olive oil until softened. Drain and add to the bowl, along with the remaining ingredients (apart from the remaining oil). Mix well.

● With lightly floured hands shape into eight burgers using the palm of your hands. Place in the fridge for 30 minutes.

● Heat the remaining 2 tablespoons of oil in a frying pan, and fry the burgers in batches for about 3 minutes on each side.

Ratatouille pasta

You can use any combination of vegetables for this dish – although the traditional ones are onions, courgettes, aubergines, tomatoes and peppers. Look at what is in season: seasonal vegetables will be cheaper and taste really good. This recipe is very quick as well, and can be prepared in advance (it improves the flavour). You can sprinkle some freshly grated Parmesan cheese over the top when serving.

SERVES 4

225g (8oz) macaroni, penne or twists (tri-colour would be fun)

For the ratatouille
3 tablespoons olive oil
1 garlic clove, peeled and crushed
350g (12oz) red or white onions, peeled and roughly diced
1 red and 1 green pepper, deseeded and roughly diced
225g (8oz) courgettes, trimmed and roughly diced
1 aubergine, trimmed and roughly diced
2 x 400g cans good Italian tomatoes
1 tablespoon tomato purée
1 teaspoon mixed dried herbs, or herbes de Provence
150ml (5fl oz) water

● Heat 1 tablespoon of the olive oil in a saucepan and gently fry the garlic and onion for about 5 minutes. Add the other 2 tablespoons of oil, along with the peppers, courgette and aubergine, and continue to cook over a moderate heat for 5 minutes.

● Add the canned tomatoes, tomato purée and herbs. Pour in the water, reduce the heat and simmer, stirring, for another 30 minutes.

● Meanwhile, in a large saucepan of boiling water, cook the pasta for 10 minutes or until tender. Drain, then mix with the vegetables. Warm through and serve.

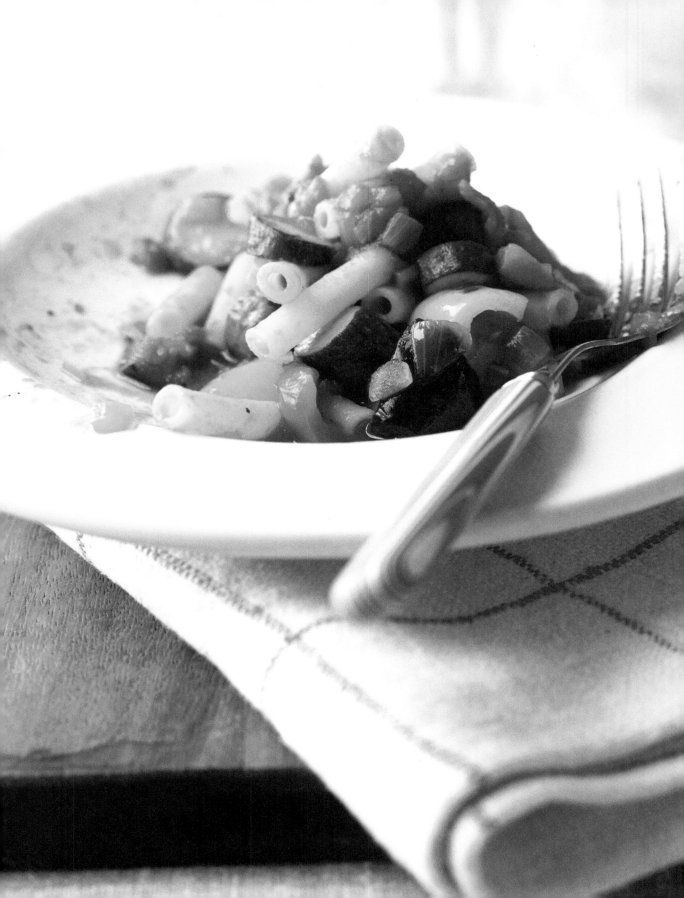

Stuffed summer vegetables

Many vegetables – cabbages, pumpkin or squashes, onions, potatoes, courgettes and aubergines – can be stuffed, but peppers and tomatoes make the most natural containers (see also the baked egg and tomato dish on page 118). You can vary the filling: if you are a meat eater, try minced meat (see page 62) instead of the rice.

SERVES 4

4 large peppers, or
   4 beef tomatoes
2 tablespoons olive oil
1 x 400g can chopped tomatoes
1 teaspoon mixed dried herbs

For the stuffing
225g (8oz) onions, peeled
   and finely chopped
1 garlic clove, peeled
   and crushed

2 tablespoons olive oil
2 tablespoons pine kernels
85g (3oz) long-grain rice
3 tablespoons finely
   chopped fresh parsley
1 tablespoon finely
   chopped fresh dill
   (or other herb of choice)
225ml (8fl oz) water

● Preheat the oven to 180°C/350°F/Gas 4.

● Cut a lid off the top of each pepper and scoop out the cores and seeds. Do the same with the tomatoes if you are using them, but drain the tomatoes upside down for a while. Keep the lids. Place in an oiled ovenproof dish.

● For the stuffing, fry the onion and garlic in the olive oil until softened and lightly coloured. Add the pine kernels, rice, herbs and water, and cook gently for 10 minutes.

● Stuff the rice mixture into the hollowed-out peppers or tomatoes to about three-quarters full (the rice will swell in cooking). Replace the lids and drizzle with the olive oil. Now take the chopped tomatoes and mix with the herbs. Pour around the stuffed vegetables and add a little water.

● Bake in the preheated oven for about 40 minutes until the vegetables are tender but are still holding their shape.

● If you like, sieve or liquidize the sauce before serving with the vegetables.

Vegetable curry

This basic curry recipe, which I begged from a colleague in Birmingham, can be varied using different vegetables from those suggested here. Serve with rice.

SERVES 4

225g (8oz) potatoes, peeled and cut into large chunks
600ml (1 pint) water or vegetable stock (see page 223)
115g (4oz) each of broccoli and cauliflower,
   cut into florets
115g (4oz) carrots, peeled and roughly chopped
115g (4oz) peas (frozen are fine)
2 tablespoons bought mild curry paste
4 tablespoons natural bio-live yoghurt

● Cook the potatoes in the water or stock for 15 minutes, then add the broccoli, cauliflower and carrots. Cook for a further 10 minutes, then add the peas and cook for 5 minutes.

● Stir in the curry paste, and combine well. Remove from the heat and allow to cool a little, then stir in the yoghurt. Serve immediately.

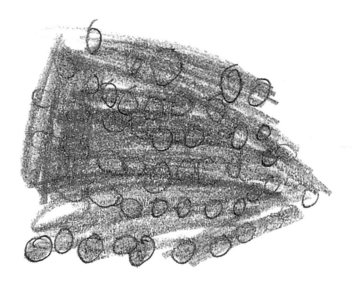

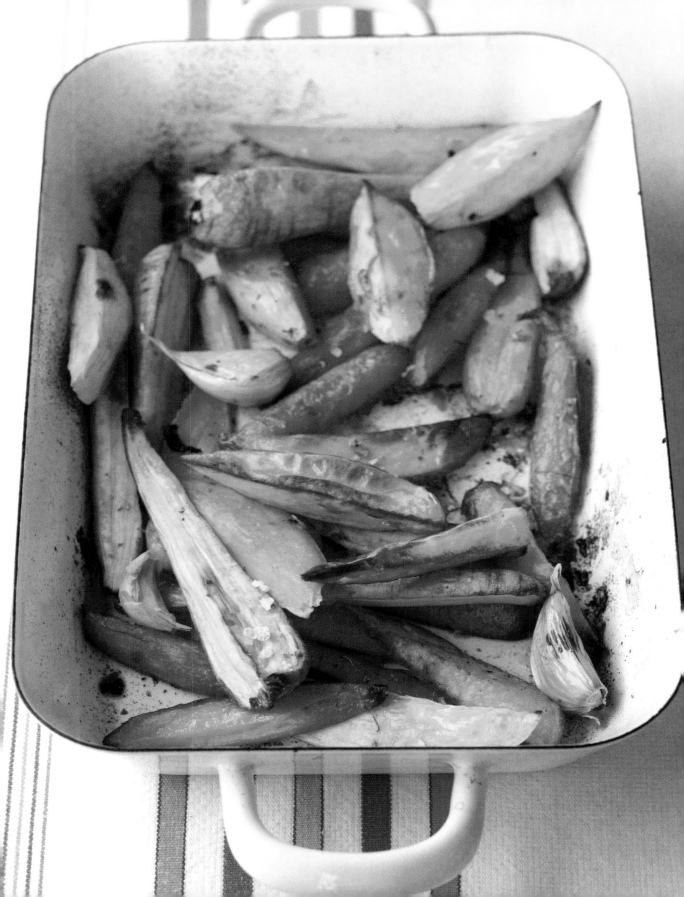

Roast vegetables

Roasting vegetables makes them sweeter somehow, and retains their essential flavour better than when they are boiled. It's difficult to be too precise about timing, but roast until the vegetables are tender, turning them occasionally if necessary.

SERVES 4

600g (1lb 5oz) vegetables (see below)
6 tablespoons olive oil
2 garlic cloves, peeled and crushed
    (and you can roast some whole too)
a few chilli flakes (optional)
1 teaspoon fresh thyme leaves, or a pinch dried

● Preheat the oven to 200°C/400°F/Gas 6.

● Prepare the vegetables. Leave young carrots, cherry tomatoes, small beetroots, scrubbed sweet potatoes, and asparagus stalks whole. Cut peeled potatoes, seeded pumpkin (skin on) and onion into good chunks. Halve or quarter parsnips, depending on size. Cut aubergines into discs about 2cm (¾in) thick. Halve sweet peppers and deseed them. Halve courgettes lengthways. Cut fennel heads in halves or thirds, depending on size.

● Mix the vegetable pieces with the remaining ingredients in a large bowl and stir to cover them with the oil and herbs. Place in an ovenproof dish or tray. Roast in the preheated oven until tender. The timing will vary according to the type and size of vegetable. In the summer, good combinations are courgettes, aubergines, tomatoes, asparagus and peppers. In the winter use pumpkin, sweet potatoes, carrots, onions and beetroot.

Vegetable (average roasting time)	
Asparagus (15 minutes)	Potatoes (45–60 minutes; new, about 30 minutes)
Aubergine discs (20–30 minutes)	
Baby beets (40 minutes)	Pumpkin (about 45–60 minutes)
Carrots/parsnips (35–40 minutes, turning once)	
Cherry tomatoes (20 minutes)	Sweet pepper, halved (about 20 minutes)
Courgettes (15 minutes)	
Fennel (30 minutes)	Sweet potatoes (45–60 minutes)
Onion (20 minutes)	

Egg-fried rice

This basic rice recipe can be expanded: try adding 115g (4oz) mushrooms, or bacon, ham or prawns if you eat fish or meat.

SERVES 4

350g (12oz) long-grain rice
2 tablespoons vegetable oil
3 eggs, beaten
2 tablespoons soy sauce
115g (4oz) frozen peas
85g (3oz) spring onions, finely sliced

● Cook the rice in boiling water until just tender (follow the instructions on the packet).

● Heat the oil in a frying pan – or a wok if you have one – and stir-fry the eggs until they begin to scramble. Add the soy sauce, peas and spring onions and lightly stir-fry for a few more minutes.

● Add the hot rice and stir-fry for 1–2 minutes or until piping hot.

Lentil rissoles

Serve in a wholemeal bun with tomato relish or soured cream. Or serve with salad and garlic bread, potato wedges or new potato salad.

SERVES 4

4 tablespoons olive oil
115g (4oz) carrots, peeled and diced
115g (4oz) onions, peeled and diced
2 celery sticks, finely diced
225g (8oz) red lentils, rinsed
½ teaspoon mixed chopped fresh herbs
500ml (18fl oz) water
25g (1oz) tomato purée
1 egg, beaten
175g (6oz) wholemeal breadcrumbs
wholemeal flour to coat

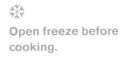

Open freeze before cooking.

● Heat half of the olive oil in a pan and sauté the vegetables until soft. Add the lentils, mixed herbs and water, bring to the boil and then simmer for 45–50 minutes, stirring occasionally. Drain off any excess water and leave to cool.

● Mix the tomato purée, beaten egg and breadcrumbs into the lentil mixture. It should be stiff. Place some wholemeal flour on a baking tray. Shape the lentil mixture into rissoles. You can use a round 7.5cm (3in) pastry cutter, or simply roll the mixture into balls and shape by hand. Coat in the flour.

● Heat the remaining olive oil in a frying pan, and cook the rissoles in batches for 10–15 minutes, turning once to brown both sides.

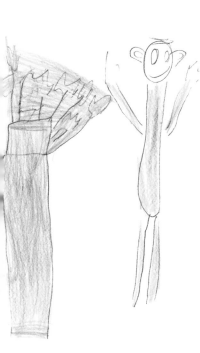

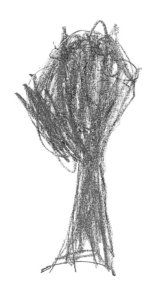

Broccoli quiche

Wholemeal pastry is good here. You can add 2 tablespoons chopped fresh parsley to the filling if you like.

SERVES 4

For the pastry
175g (6oz) wholemeal flour
55g (2oz) plain flour
55g (2oz) butter, cut into cubes
55g (2oz) vegetable shortening, cut into cubes
2 tablespoons water

For the filling
450g (1lb) broccoli, cut into small florets
225g (8oz) spring onion
olive oil
6 eggs
225ml (8fl oz) milk
280g (10oz) Cheddar cheese, grated
1 tablespoon sesame seeds (optional)

This quiche and the flan opposite can be frozen after cooking. You could also freeze the empty pastry case, ready for use at a future date.

● Make and blind bake a pastry case as described on page 66, in a 25 x 20cm (10 x 8in) solid-bottomed flan tin.

● Preheat the oven to 190°C/375°F/Gas 5.

● Blanch the broccoli in boiling water for 2–3 minutes, then drain well. Cut the green of the spring onion into 5mm (¼in) lengths, and finely slice the remaining white onion. Stir-fry the spring onion in a little olive oil for about 1–2 minutes. Beat the eggs and milk together.

● Place the spring onion and broccoli in the part-baked pastry case, and sprinkle with the grated cheese. Pour the eggs and milk through a sieve over the broccoli. Sprinkle with sesame seeds if liked. Bake in the preheated oven for 30–35 minutes until golden brown and set.

Cheese and lentil flan

Lentils are highly nutritious, and, cooked with cheese, onion and eggs, they are deliciously savoury.

SERVES 4

For the pastry
225g (8oz) plain flour
55g (2oz) butter, cut into cubes
55g (2oz) vegetable shortening, cut into cubes
2 tablespoons water

For the filling
115g (4oz) red lentils, washed
115g (4oz) red onion, peeled and sliced
1 tablespoon olive oil
3 eggs
200ml (7fl oz) milk
280g (10oz) Cheddar cheese, grated
1 tablespoon chopped fresh chives

● Make and blind bake a pastry case as described on page 66, in a 25 x 20cm (10 x 8in) solid-bottomed flan tin.

● Preheat the oven to 190°C/375°F/Gas 5.

● To make the filling, bring the lentils to the boil in plenty of water, then simmer for 25–35 minutes until soft. Drain very well.

● Fry the onion in the olive oil until soft, about 5–10 minutes. Beat the eggs with the milk.

● Combine the lentils and onion and place in the bottom of the flan case. Sprinkle the grated cheese and chives over the lentils and onions. Carefully strain the egg and milk through a sieve over the cheese, making sure it is completely covered. Bake in the preheated oven for 30–35 minutes until the filling is golden brown and set.

Broccoli and cherry tomato cheese

If your children don't like anything green, they may like this because of the sweetness of the cherry tomatoes. For a more sophisticated flavour, make the sauce using Stilton, my local cheese.

SERVES 4

450g (1lb) broccoli, cut into florets
225g (8oz) cherry tomatoes (the vine ones are nice), washed
25g (1oz) butter
25g (1oz) plain flour
600ml (1 pint) milk
1 tablespoon wholegrain mustard
225g (8oz) Cheddar cheese, grated

● Preheat the oven to 200°C/400°F/Gas 6.

● Wash the broccoli florets in cold water, then cook in boiling water for 5–10 minutes. Drain well and place in an ovenproof dish. Arrange the cherry tomatoes in the dish.

● To make the cheese sauce, melt the butter in a small pan, then add the flour, and cook until the texture and colour are sandy. Add the milk and stir continuously until thickened and smooth. Add the mustard and most of the cheese (reserving some for the top), and remove from the heat.

● Pour the sauce over the broccoli and tomatoes, sprinkle the remaining cheese over the top, and bake in the preheated oven for 10 minutes or until the cheese has melted and browned.

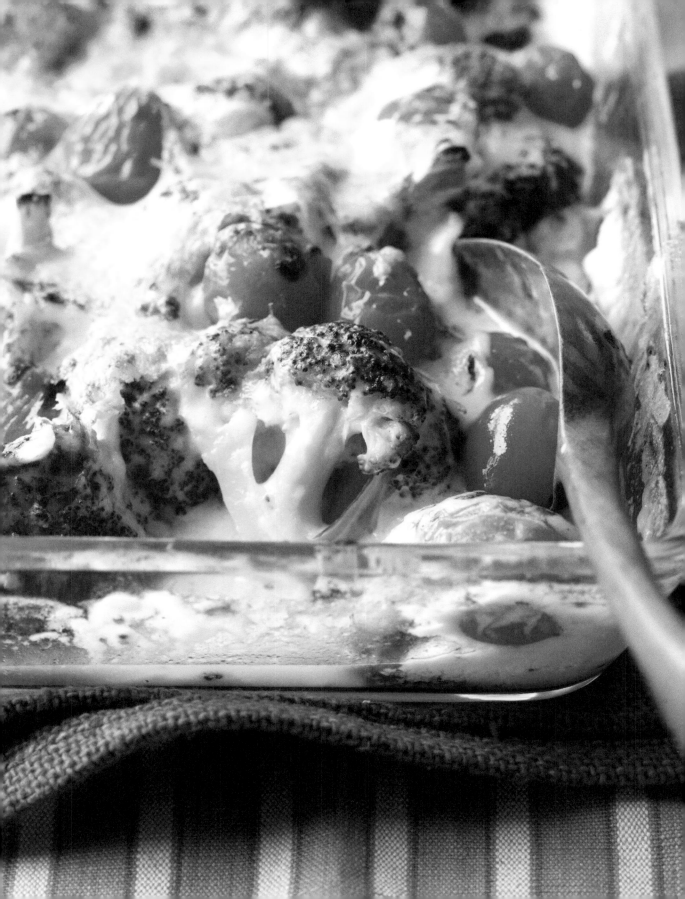

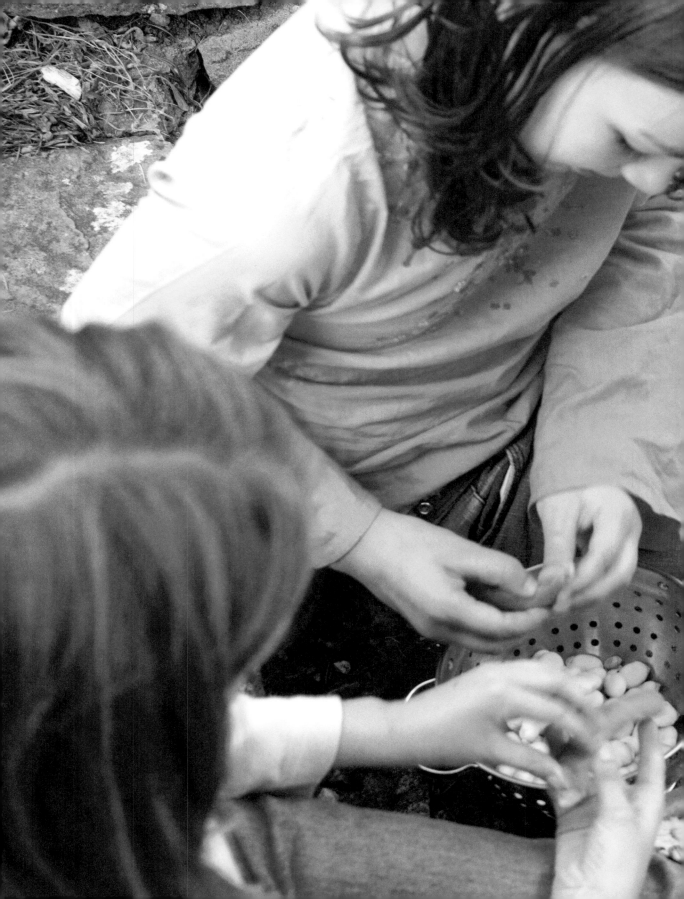

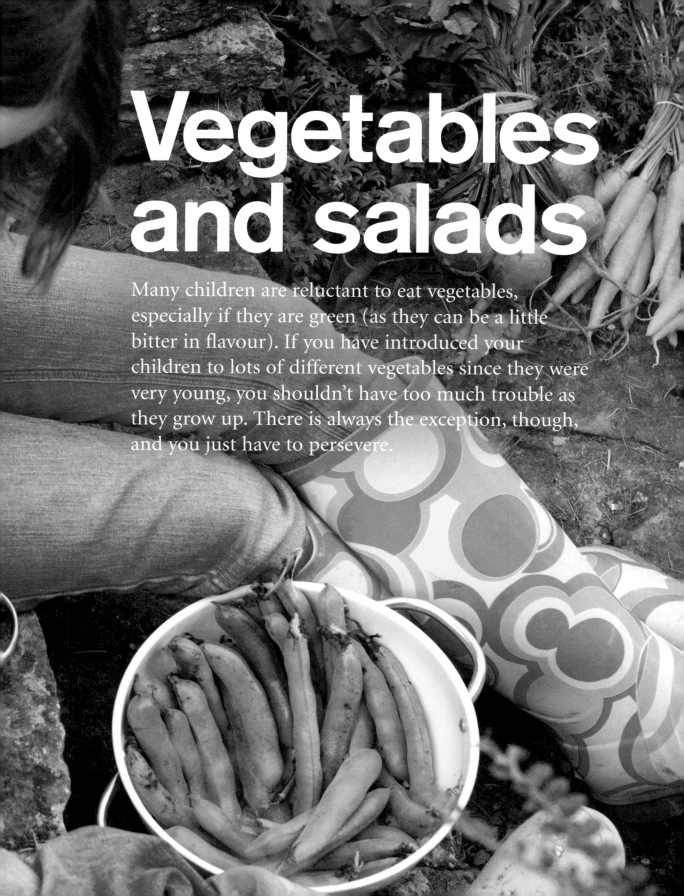

Vegetables and salads

Many children are reluctant to eat vegetables, especially if they are green (as they can be a little bitter in flavour). If you have introduced your children to lots of different vegetables since they were very young, you shouldn't have too much trouble as they grow up. There is always the exception, though, and you just have to persevere.

TRY BRIGHTLY COLOURED VEGETABLES (yellow, orange and green vegetables are the most nutritious), cut them small (if necessary) and cook them so that they are neither too soft nor too hard, or just serve them raw (see page 71)! Try different combinations of vegetables, and stir-fry or bake them perhaps, instead of boiling.

I've divided this section up into two parts. The first part deals with potatoes, which children love – and there is not a chip in sight – and other vegetables, followed by a second part on salads and dressings.

Jacket potatoes are good simply baked for an hour or so, depending on size, and topped with baked beans or grated cheese (a firm and continuing favourite at St Peter's). There is a new baked potato idea here, which all the children I've tested it on have loved, and I've also baked sweet potato in wedges. But potatoes can be baked in other ways, in layers with protein-rich cheese and/or milk, and with vegetables. They're good as supper dishes, or accompaniments to meats and fish.

Mashed potato is another favourite, and there are a few ideas here for adding extra flavour, or toppings. If your children like the texture of mash, they may also take to other vegetable mashes, such as parsnip, carrot or pumpkin, too.

Some vegetables you don't have to cook, because you can serve them as salads. You can make them the night before, pop them in an airtight plastic box, and store in the fridge. Salads containing raw vegetables and fruit, with perhaps some cheese or nuts, or cooked rice or potato, are important. They look good, taste good, and can do your children – and you – good!

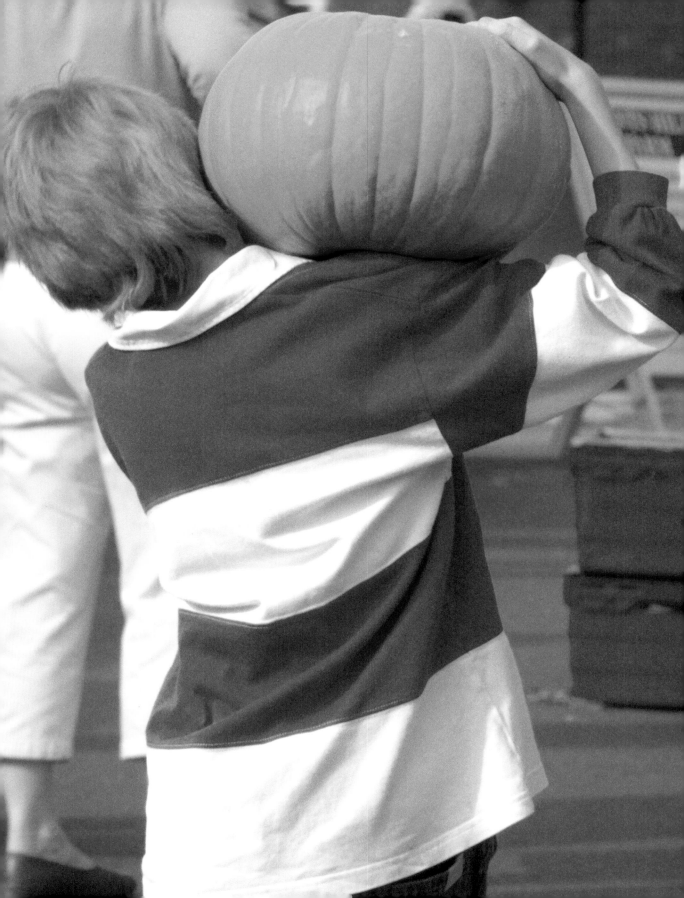

Mashed potato

There is nothing like a good mash, and potatoes provide essential carbohydrates. You don't have to add anything apart from a little milk and butter, but you can also 'spice' them up (see below for a few ideas).

Some people use a fork to mash potatoes, others use a potato masher or a potato ricer. I went to stay with a friend in Norfolk and she used a mouli, and I must say the potatoes were delicious. Whichever way you do it, mash the potatoes before you add the flavouring. A good tip is to warm the milk before adding it, as this will keep the potatoes nice and hot.

Some potatoes, depending on variety, will need more or less milk, so add a little at a time.

SERVES 4

450g (1lb) potatoes, peeled and quartered
3–4 tablespoons milk
25–40g (1–1½ oz) butter

● Put the potatoes in a large pan, cover with water, bring to the boil and simmer for 20–25 minutes until a skewer goes easily through the middle of the potato. Drain well.

● Mash the potato, then add the milk gradually and mash again. Add half of the butter and mash again. If needed, add the remaining butter, mash again, and serve.

Variations

Some people like blue cheese in their potato, others prefer pesto. Try adding some roasted garlic (to taste!) or a teaspoon of creamed horseradish. The Irish mix cooked onion and cabbage with mashed potato, in a delicious recipe called 'colcannon' or 'champ', and that's what I do for my version of bubble and squeak (see page 196). Try one of the following ideas, or you can make one up yourself.

● 1 teaspoon wholegrain mustard

● 1 teaspoon chopped fresh chives

● 55g (2oz) cheese, grated

● 25g (1oz) cream cheese

● 55g (2oz) red onion, diced very finely then cooked

Lyonnaise potatoes

This is a great way to serve potatoes, especially with a roast, for a change. You could use milk instead of the stock, which makes the potatoes slightly richer. If you have one, use a mandolin to slice the potatoes and onions; it's much easier!

SERVES 4

40g (1½ oz) butter, chopped into knobs
1kg (2¼ lb) old potatoes, peeled and very thinly sliced
175g (6oz) onions, peeled and very thinly sliced
1 teaspoon chopped fresh rosemary
   or thyme, or 1 teaspoon dried
600ml (1 pint) vegetable stock (see page 223)
25g (1oz) Cheddar cheese, grated (optional)

● Preheat the oven to 180°C/350°F/Gas 4. Use about 15g (½oz) of the butter to grease a 1.5 litre (2¾ pint) ovenproof dish.

● Layer the potatoes and onions in the prepared dish, finishing with a layer of potato. Add the herbs. Pour over the vegetable stock and place knobs of butter on the top. Sprinkle with the cheese, if using.

● Cover with foil and bake in the preheated oven for 30 minutes. Remove the foil and return to the oven for another 15 minutes or so until light brown on the top, and the potatoes are soft.

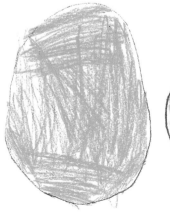
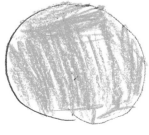

My bubble and squeak

This used to be made with Sunday lunch leftovers on a Monday for a quick supper. It is great with the lamb burgers on page 131 and the tomato salsa on page 230. The mixture is quite hard to shape, but it's worth persevering because it tastes wonderful!

SERVES 4

450g (1lb) old potatoes, peeled and diced
50ml (2fl oz) milk
55g (2oz) butter
225g (8oz) green cabbage, finely shredded
2 tablespoons olive oil

These freeze very well once cooked.

● Cook the potatoes in boiling water for 15–20 minutes until tender, then drain. Mash with the milk and half the butter, then put to one side to cool.

● Cook the cabbage in a saucepan of boiling water for 3–5 minutes only, then drain well. Mix the cabbage into the potato mixture, and leave until cool enough to handle.

● With floured hands make eight potato cakes. Heat the remaining butter and the olive oil in a frying pan. Add the cakes and fry for about 2–3 minutes on each side, until golden brown and warmed through.

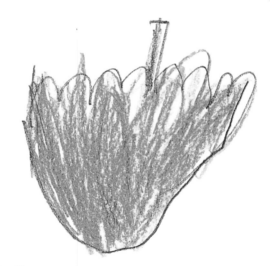

Cheesy potato bake

This could be served on its own in small dishes for a vegetarian meal, or as an accompaniment to a meat dish. You could add some meat to make it a main dish: try 115g (4oz) chopped ham. It can be prepared ahead.

SERVES 4

450g (1lb) old potatoes, peeled and cut into thick slices
    (about 2.5cm/1in)
vegetable oil
225g (8oz) leeks, washed and cut into 1cm (½in) chunks
1 tablespoon chopped fresh chives

For the cheese sauce
25g (1oz) butter
25g (1oz) plain flour
600ml (1 pint) milk
115g (4oz) Cheddar or other hard cheese, grated

● Preheat the oven to 200°C/400°F/Gas 6.

● Blanch the potato slices in boiling water for 2–3 minutes, then drain well. In a lightly oiled ovenproof dish, layer the potato and leek slices alternately. Sprinkle the fresh chives over the layers.

● To make the sauce, melt the butter in a saucepan and add the flour. Cook until sandy in texture, then add the milk and cook, stirring for 5–10 minutes until thickened. Add nearly all the cheese, saving some for the top. When the cheese has melted, pour the sauce over the potatoes and leeks. Sprinkle with the remaining cheese.

● Bake in the preheated oven for 25–30 minutes until golden brown and cooked through.

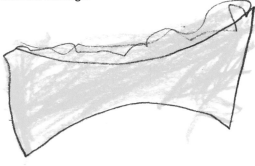

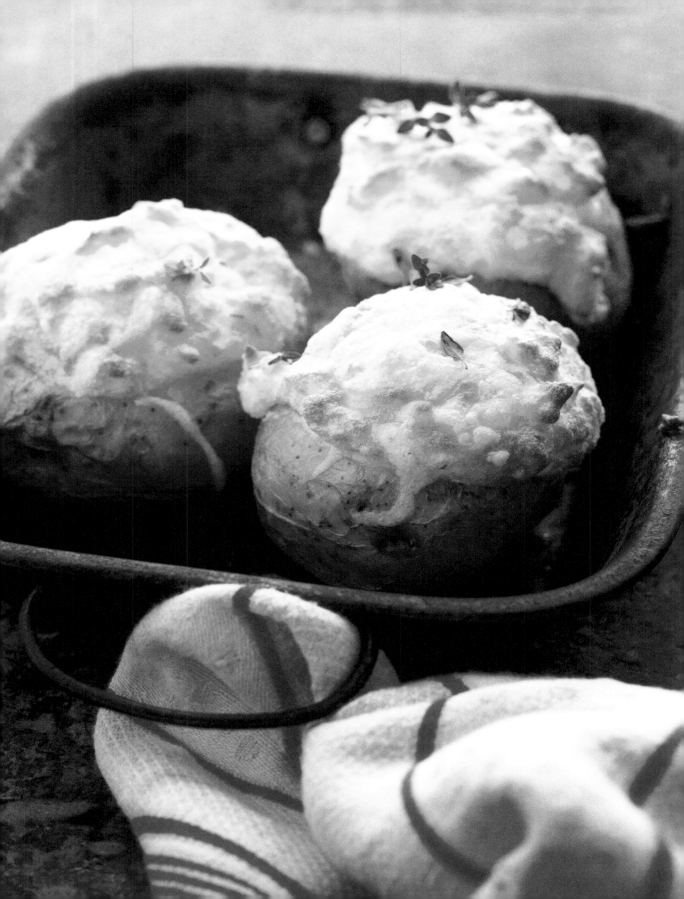

Baked soufflé potatoes

All children like baked potatoes, and this is a slightly different way of presenting them – with the added goodness of eggs. The potato flesh is enriched with egg yolks and whipped egg whites, and baked to a soufflé texture in the potato skins. You can use different flavourings – a blue cheese, for instance, some pesto (see page 232), or top with some crispy bacon bits.

SERVES 4

2 large baking potatoes, about 350g (12oz) each, washed
25g (1oz) butter
1 teaspoon freshly grated nutmeg
½ teaspoon English mustard
3 medium eggs, separated
55g (2oz) Cheddar cheese, finely grated
a few fresh thyme leaves

● Preheat the oven to 190°C/375°F/Gas 5.

● Bake the potatoes in the preheated oven until tender, about 1–1½ hours, depending on size. Once they have cooled slightly, halve them lengthways. Keeping the potato skins whole to use as containers, use a spoon to carefully scoop out the flesh and set it to one side. Put the potato skins in an ovenproof dish.

● Mash the potato flesh with the butter, nutmeg, mustard, egg yolks and cheese. Whisk the egg whites in a separate bowl until stiff, and then stir a couple of tablespoons into the potato mixture. Fold in the remaining egg white using a metal spoon, trying to keep as much 'airiness' as possible.

● Turn the oven temperature up to 200°C/400°F/Gas 6. Spoon the soufflé mixture back into the potato skins, and return to the oven for about 15 minutes until the potato soufflés have risen and become golden brown, and the skins are crisp. Sprinkle with the thyme.

Sweet potato wedges with spicy yoghurt

You can use ordinary potatoes for this recipe though they may need to be cooked for a little longer, as sweet potatoes have softer flesh. Serve with any of the traditional baked potato accompaniments – melted butter or soured cream, or the yoghurt mix below. Some of the dips on pages 229–35 would be good, especially the cucumber and yoghurt.

SERVES 4

675g (1½lb) sweet potatoes, scrubbed
2 tablespoons olive oil
1 tablespoon soy sauce

For the spicy yoghurt
300ml (10fl oz) natural bio-live yoghurt
½ teaspoon ground cumin or garam masala
½ red chilli, deseeded and very finely chopped
juice and finely grated rind of 1 lime
a handful of fresh coriander leaves, chopped

● Preheat the oven to 200°C/400°F/Gas 6.

● Dry the sweet potatoes and peel them if you like (although they hold their shape better if the skin is still on). Cut lengthwise into quarters. Put in an ovenproof dish in one layer, and pour in the olive oil and soy sauce. Toss carefully so that the potato wedges are evenly coated. Bake in the preheated oven for 25 minutes until golden and crisp.

● For the spicy yoghurt, simply mix everything together, going easy on the juice if it looks as if it is getting too thin.

● Serve the potato wedges hot, with a dollop of the spicy yoghurt at the side.

Vegetable mashes

Kids love mashed potato, but you can do the same with many other vegetables, or even a mixture of potato and another vegetable. You can make a basic mash with all the root vegetables − carrots, parsnips, onions, Jerusalem artichokes, swedes (what the Scots call 'neeps', and eat with their haggis), sweet potatoes, celeriac and turnips − and you can also use pumpkin or squash (roast them first rather than boil, see page 182), Brussels sprouts, broccoli and cauliflower.

SERVES 4

450g (1lb) chosen vegetable (or a mixture), peeled and trimmed
15g (½oz) butter
milk (optional)
flavouring or topping to taste (see below)

● Prepare the vegetables as appropriate. Steam (this is slightly healthier, as it retains more nutrients) over boiling water, or cook in boiling water, until tender. If you are steaming, put the harder vegetables under the other vegetables because they take longer. Drain very well. Dry out a little in the pan over a low heat. Add the butter and mash until smooth either with a potato masher or by pushing the vegetables through a sieve or blitzing them in a blender or processor (the latter isn't good with potatoes). If the mash is very dry, add a little milk to taste, or a little more butter.

Vegetable purée toppings and flavourings

● Toasted sunflower seeds, sesame seeds, pine kernels or chopped nuts (if there is no nut allergy involved).

● Shreds of crispy bacon.

● A colour contrast, such as tiny squares of red pepper on a white mash.

● Finely grated citrus rind (orange is good with carrot).

● Coarsely ground black pepper looks and tastes good on many mashes.

● Chopped or torn soft-leaved herbs sprinkled on top, for instance coriander with carrot, and chervil or parsley with almost anything.

● Ground spice such as nutmeg or coriander sprinkled on top, or incorporated while mashing.

● Cheese added to the more unusual mashes will make them more appealing to children.

Braised peas, lettuce and spring onions

A different idea for peas, and a great way of using up lettuces when you have too many in your garden! It's delicious served with grilled or roast meat or fish.

SERVES 4

55g (2oz) butter
1 round soft lettuce, about 225g (8oz), shredded
4 large spring onions, both white and green parts,
    trimmed and chopped
3 tablespoons chopped fresh mint (or a mixture, e.g. parsley, basil,
    mint, chives)
450g (1lb) frozen petits pois

● Melt the butter in a saucepan. Add the lettuce and onion and gently cook – it's known as 'sweating' – for about 5 minutes until softened.

● Add the herbs and peas and a little water – about 50ml (2fl oz) – and cover with the lid. Stew gently for about 20 minutes.

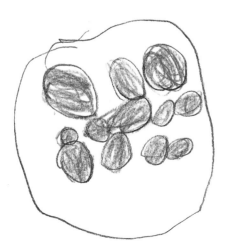

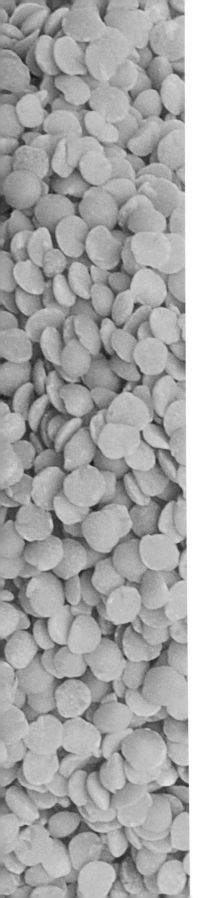

Red lentil dhal

Serve as an accompaniment to meat or curries, perhaps with rice. The cooking fat traditionally used is ghee, which is a clarified butter (often made from buffalo milk). Olive oil is a little healthier.

SERVES 4

225g (8oz) red lentils
175g (6oz) onions, peeled and finely diced
1 garlic clove, peeled and crushed
2 tablespoons olive oil
½ teaspoon turmeric
½ teaspoon ground ginger
½ teaspoon chilli powder
1 teaspoon ground cumin
850ml (1½ pints) water
1 lemon, cut into slices
1 cinnamon stick
a knob of butter (optional)

● Rinse the lentils and wash and drain them.

● Sauté the onion and garlic in the olive oil in a medium saucepan for a few minutes, then add the ground spices and stir well. Cook gently for 5 minutes.

● Add the water, lentils, sliced lemon and cinnamon stick. Cover the pan and simmer for 40 minutes or until the lentils are tender. Remove the lemon and cinnamon just before serving. If you like, stir in the butter to enrich the flavour.

Courgette, potato and cheese layer

Adding yoghurt to the white sauce here really lightens the dish. You can assemble this in advance, and chill until ready to cook it.

SERVES 4

450g (1lb) old potatoes, peeled and sliced
350g (12oz) courgettes, trimmed and cut into slices 1cm (½in) thick
25g (1oz) butter, plus a little extra for greasing
175g (6oz) onions, peeled and sliced
1 garlic clove, peeled and finely chopped
225g (8oz) cherry tomatoes, halved
115g (4oz) wholemeal breadcrumbs

For the yoghurt cheese sauce
25g (1oz) butter
25g (1oz) plain flour
300ml (10fl oz) milk
200g (7oz) Cheddar cheese, coarsely grated
280g (10oz) natural bio-live yoghurt

● Preheat the oven to 170°C/325°F/Gas 3.

● Blanch the potatoes in a pan of boiling water for 5 minutes. Remove with a slotted spoon. Then blanch the courgettes in the same boiling water for about 2 minutes, and drain.

● Melt the butter in a frying pan, and cook the onion and garlic until soft, about 5 minutes.

● To make the sauce, melt the butter in a pan, add the flour and cook for 2–3 minutes, stirring all the time, until sandy in colour. Stir in the milk and cook until thick. Add 140g (5oz) of the cheese, reserving the rest for the top. Stir until the cheese has melted, then stir in the yoghurt.

● In a greased ovenproof dish, begin with a layer of potato. Add a layer of courgette, then scatter evenly with some of the cherry tomato halves, the fried onion and garlic, and a little of the sauce. Continue building the layers, which don't need to be neat, finishing with the potatoes. Pour over the remaining sauce and sprinkle with the breadcrumbs, then the reserved cheese. Bake for 40–45 minutes until bubbling.

Vegetable rösti

This is a Swiss recipe usually made with only potato, but I have added a few other vegetables as well.

SERVES 4

350g (12oz) courgettes, washed
350g (12oz) carrots, peeled
115g (4oz) parsnips, peeled
225g (8oz) old potatoes, peeled
1 egg, beaten
1 tablespoon plain flour
2 tablespoons olive oil

These freeze well after cooking. Defrost and reheat in a low oven before serving.

● Grate the courgette on to paper towel and squeeze out any excess water. Put into a mixing bowl. Grate and drain the carrot, parsnip and potato the same way, then combine them all in the mixing bowl. Add the beaten egg and flour, and mix well.

● Heat the oil over a medium heat in a large frying pan. Divide the mixture into eight pieces of about a tablespoonful each. Put them in the pan in batches that will fit your pan, and flatten them down with a fish slice. Cook for 3–4 minutes on each side until golden brown.

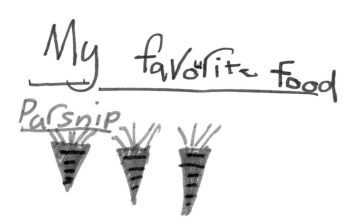

My favourite food
Parsnip

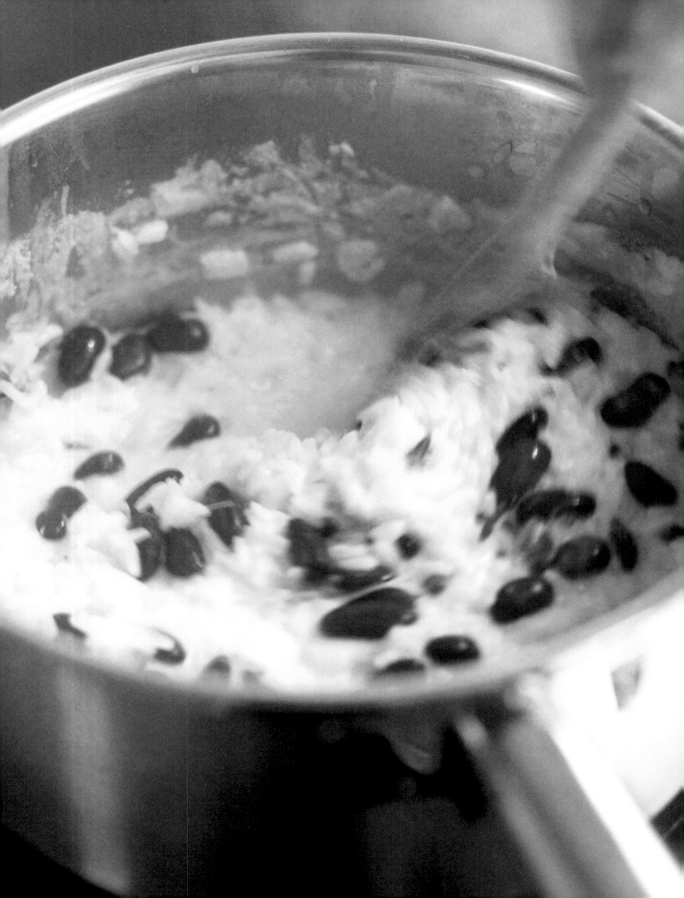

Caribbean rice and peas

In the West Indies, beans or pulses are known as 'peas', and so here we are using red kidney beans. This recipe was given to me by a friend who cooks at a school in South London. She says it is great served with a spicy Jamaican chicken dish (you can buy Jamaican spices in jars).

SERVES 4

vegetable oil
175g (6oz) onions, peeled and finely chopped
2 garlic cloves, peeled and finely chopped
a few chilli flakes (optional)
175g (6oz) long-grain rice
450ml (15fl oz) coconut milk
1 teaspoon fresh thyme leaves
2 x 400g cans red kidney beans, rinsed and drained

● Preheat the oven to 200°C/400°F/Gas 6.

● Heat the oil in a large pan and fry the onion, garlic and chilli, if using, until soft, about 5–10 minutes. Add the rice and fry for about a minute.

● Put the coconut milk and thyme in a measuring jug, and add 200ml (7fl oz) water. Add to the rice along with the beans, cover and bring to the boil.

● Transfer the mixture to an ovenproof dish, cover and cook in the preheated oven for 15–20 minutes.

salads

Spinach, bacon and apple salad

Some children do not like spinach as it has a strong flavour; try to find baby leaves, as they will be sweeter. Or you can use cos or baby gem lettuce instead. And of course some children will not like the nuts – or may have allergies – so they are optional although they add an interesting crunch.

SERVES 4

225g (8oz) fresh baby spinach leaves, washed and dried
175g (6oz) smoked bacon rashers, rinded and diced
2 Granny Smith apples, cored and finely diced
a handful of walnut halves (optional)
about 115g (4oz) feta cheese, cut into small chunks (optional)
1 tablespoon olive oil

● Tear away any coarse spinach stems. Shred the leaves, and place in a bowl or on individual plates.

● Fry the diced bacon in a dry pan until brown and crisp. Add the apple and walnuts (if using) and stir-fry for a minute or so. Pour the contents of the pan, including the bacon fat, over the spinach, sprinkle in the cheese (if using) and olive oil, and toss.

Celery and apple salad

Good fresh walnuts add flavour to this crispy salad, but you could use other nuts (if there is no nut allergy) such as almonds, hazelnuts, pecans or pine kernels. Toast them first to add another element of flavour. Serve this with barbecued meats, or fish. You can add some cos or gem lettuce if you like.

SERVES 4

1 small head fresh celery, about 350g (12oz), washed and trimmed
4 medium red or russet apples, about 350g (12oz),
   washed, quartered and cored
2 tablespoons vinaigrette (see page 217)
3 tablespoons mayonnaise (see page 216)
55g (2oz) walnut halves, chopped (optional)
a small bunch of watercress, rinsed

● Separate the celery into sticks and slice them into very fine half-moons. Finely slice the cored apple quarters and put in a bowl with the celery. Pour over the vinaigrette and mix. Add the mayonnaise and combine.

● Just before serving, chop the walnuts and mix them into the salad. Place the salad in a bowl, or on individual plates, and top with sprigs of watercress.

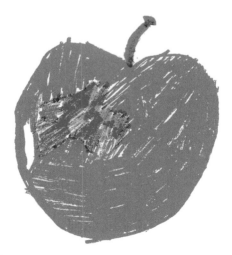

Cucumber and strawberry salad

In the summer, if you have grown, bought or picked a glut of strawberries, try incorporating them into a salad instead of just serving them as a pudding. Their sweet softness contrasts with the crisp tang of the cucumber here. Serve with fish, cold chicken or turkey.

SERVES 4

350g (12oz) cucumber, washed and halved lengthways
280g (10oz) strawberries, wiped and hulled
sprinkling of fresh herbs (parsley or basil, perhaps), chopped
2 tablespoons vinaigrette (see page 217)

● Use a teaspoon to remove the seeds from both halves of the cucumber. Finely slice the halves into half-moons.

● Cut the strawberries into thin slices. Arrange the cucumber and strawberry slices in a pattern, or haphazardly if you like, on a dish or plate. Sprinkle with the herbs and vinaigrette.

● Chill before serving.

Tomato, avocado and mozzarella salad

This is a classic Italian salad, utilizing all the colours of the Italian flag. It is also delicious, and very good for you. If the children like its taste, you could substitute the Greek feta cheese for the mozzarella, but that is far from traditional! Instead of slicing everything, you can cut into small chunks as in the photograph. You can make this salad up to 2 hours in advance.

SERVES 4

2 large tomatoes, washed and finely sliced
1 ripe avocado, halved with stone removed
1 x 150g packet mozzarella cheese, drained and thinly sliced
a handful of fresh basil leaves, rinsed and dried
2 tablespoons vinaigrette (see page 217)

● Arrange the tomatoes in a serving dish. Peel the avocado halves and then slice the flesh finely. Arrange the avocado and mozzarella cheese slices decoratively (or haphazardly) with the tomato slices. Sprinkle with the basil and the vinaigrette.

● Chill before serving.

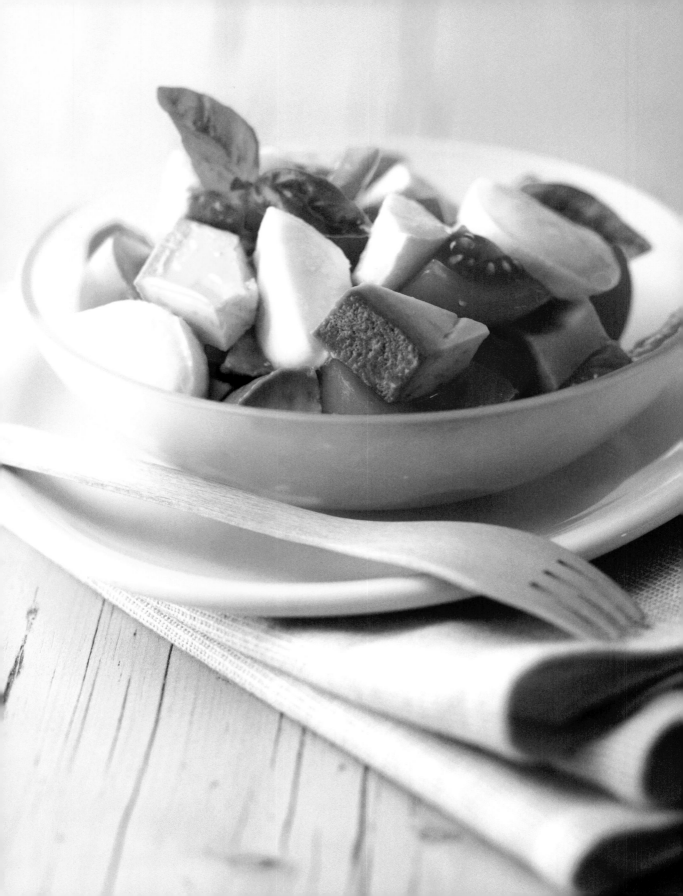

Brown rice salad

This can be eaten by itself or as an accompaniment to other salads or cold meats. You can make this salad with white long-grain rice if you prefer (cook for 10 minutes less), but brown is healthier. If spiced up a bit, the salad could be served with curry-type meals (turmeric would colour the rice yellow). Don't feel you have to follow the instructions below to the letter, as basically anything can be mixed into a rice salad – finely chopped vegetables, shreds of cooked leftover meat, ham or cooked poultry, other dried fruits, and nuts and seeds. Use your imagination!

SERVES 4

200g (7oz) brown rice
1 x 400g can red kidney beans, rinsed and drained
125ml (4fl oz) vinaigrette (see page 217)
40g (1½oz) raisins or sultanas
40g (1½ oz) dried apricots, finely chopped
55g (2oz) walnut halves, coarsely chopped
2 tablespoons chopped fresh basil

● Cook the rice in boiling water for about 30–35 minutes, then drain very well. While still warm mix the rice with all the other ingredients. Leave to cool, then chill.

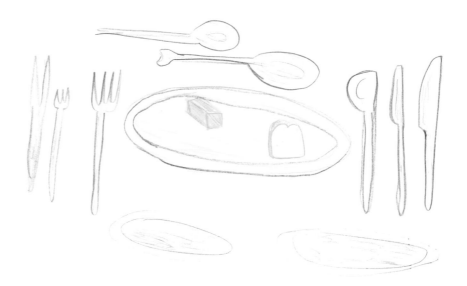

Potato salad

If you prefer a lighter dressing, use 3 tablespoons each of natural bio-live yoghurt and mayonnaise.

SERVES 4

450g (1lb) new potatoes
175g (6oz) mayonnaise (see page 216)

● Scrub the potatoes (you don't have to get all the skin off), and cut in half if large. Simmer for 15–20 minutes, until just soft, then drain and put in a serving bowl.

● Add the mayonnaise while the potatoes are still warm, combining carefully so as not to break them up. Stir in any variations now (see below).

Variations

You can also add the following:

● 2 spring onions, finely chopped

● 225g (8oz) frozen sweetcorn, cooked

● 175g (6oz) red onion, finely diced

● 1 hard-boiled egg, chopped

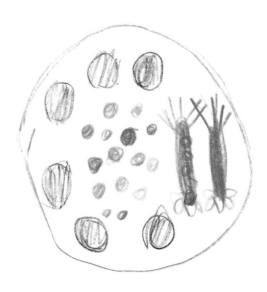

Mayonnaise

Making mayonnaise by hand is a laborious process, but once you get the hang of it, it's easy. In fact I find it quite relaxing, and it's very satisfactory seeing the eggs and oil gradually transformed into a rich and thick dressing. You can use a balloon whisk, or an electric hand whisk. Or, of course, you can make the mayonnaise completely in the food processor. As it takes time, it is worth making a fairly large amount; it will last for a couple of days in the fridge. You can also ring the changes, and make different types of mayonnaise (see below).

MAKES 350ml (12fl oz)

2 egg yolks
2 tablespoons white wine vinegar or 1 tablespoon lemon juice
1 teaspoon Dijon mustard
300ml (10fl oz) vegetable or olive oil (or a mixture – some olive
    oils make quite a strong mayonnaise)

● In a small bowl set on a tea-towel on the work surface, whisk the egg yolks with half the vinegar or lemon juice and the mustard until thick.

● Add the oil, drop by drop at first, constantly whisking. After adding about 2–3 tablespoons in this very gradual fashion, start adding it more swiftly, in a slow stream, still whisking constantly. Once all the oil has been whisked in and the mayonnaise is thick, stir in the remaining vinegar or lemon juice. Taste and add more vinegar, lemon juice or mustard if needed.

Variations

● **Aïoli** is a garlic mayonnaise, good with fish, eggs and vegetables. Crush as many peeled garlic cloves as you dare, and add to the basic recipe instead of the mustard. Roasting the garlic first makes a mellower flavour. (Bake for 25 minutes in a moderate oven, then squeeze out the cloves into the mayo.)

● To make a **green mayonnaise** for fish, eggs and vegetables, stir in either finely chopped fresh herbs or some puréed cooked spinach.

● To make a **tomato mayonnaise**, add 1–2 tablespoons tomato ketchup or tomato purée. This is also known as Marie Rose sauce, and it is used in prawn cocktail.

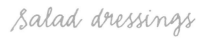
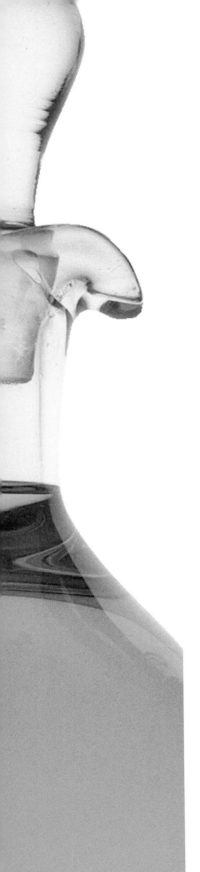

● **Tartare sauce**, which goes so well with fish, is based on mayonnaise. Add some chopped hard-boiled egg whites, and chopped capers, gherkins, shallot and parsley.

● Dill is a taste many children like, and a **dill and mustard sauce** is a good accompaniment to fish and many cold meats. Stir 3 tablespoons Dijon or English mustard into the mayonnaise, along with about 3 tablespoons chopped fresh dill.

Vinaigrette

Also known as French dressing, this is an ideal dressing for salads. You can vary it in a number of ways. Adding fresh chopped herbs (about 2 tablespoons) makes a delicious herb dressing for a pasta, rice or potato salad; you could also add crushed garlic. Simply using different oils (olive, sunflower, walnut or a mixture) or vinegars (red or white wine and fruit vinegars are good) gives each dressing its own character. You could also try using different mustards: a grain mustard dressing is interesting.

MAKES 125ml (4fl oz)

2 tablespoons wine or cider vinegar (never malt), or
   1½ tablespoons lemon juice
1 teaspoon English or Dijon mustard (depending on how hot you
   like it; it is entirely optional)
6 tablespoons olive oil (or, lighter, a mix of sunflower and olive)

● In a small bowl whisk the wine vinegar or lemon juice with the mustard if using. Gradually add the oil, whisking constantly, until the two liquids come together, or emulsify. Or you could simply put all the ingredients into a small screw-top jar and shake them together. Keep in the fridge. This is particularly handy in the summer, when salads are eaten more often.

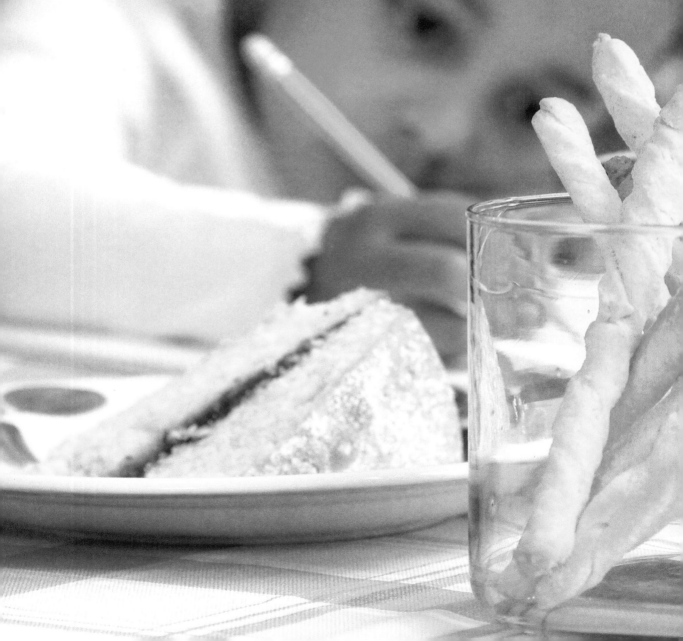

Home from school

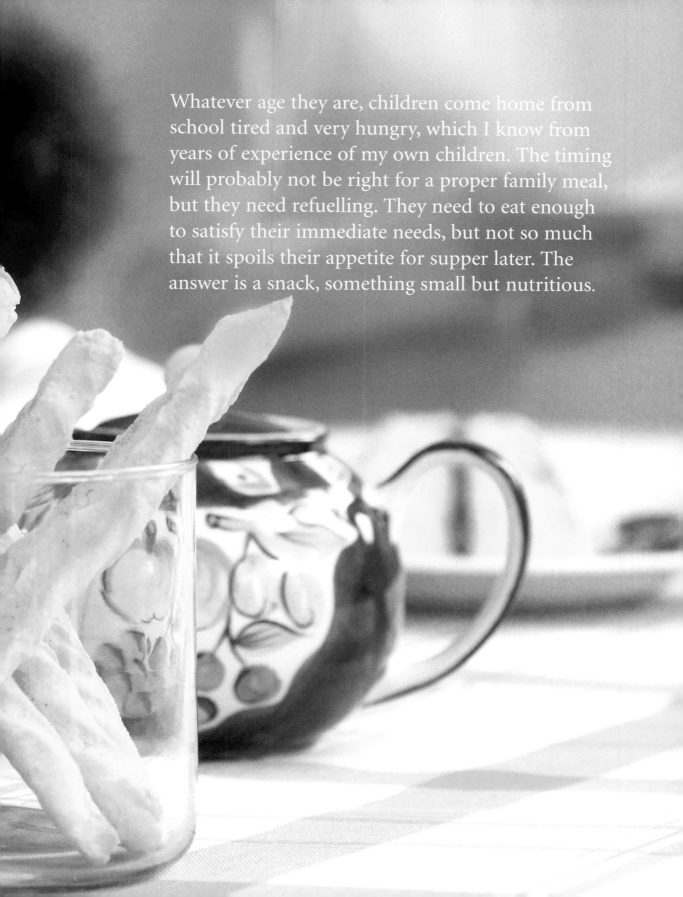

Whatever age they are, children come home from school tired and very hungry, which I know from years of experience of my own children. The timing will probably not be right for a proper family meal, but they need refuelling. They need to eat enough to satisfy their immediate needs, but not so much that it spoils their appetite for supper later. The answer is a snack, something small but nutritious.

'SNACK' IS AN UNFORTUNATE WORD these days, as it immediately suggests crisps, chips, biscuits, chocolate or cake, which should be limited in any child's diet. Indeed too much snacking, or eating between meals, is not a good idea in general. Children 'graze' too much these days, which can make them less receptive to food at proper mealtimes. But there are times when something is needed – particularly for very young children, whose stomachs are small – and there are plenty of healthy foods that would be a better alternative. Fruit, either fresh or dried, is probably the best snack, perhaps with a handful of unsalted nuts. Young children home from playgroup or nursery may be satisfied with a nutritious drink (see the Breakfasts section for some ideas), and older children might appreciate a mug of soup with a roll or piece of bread – there are lots of soups on page 224. Another easy filler is a dip or spread, with chunks of raw vegetables to dip into them: I used to give this to my boys when they came home, and it kept them going until it was time for their evening meal. You can use a variety of other things to dip: toasted ordinary or pitta bread, bought nachos or tortilla chips, or the Melba toast or breadsticks on pages 245 and 246. In fact many of the dips on pages 229–35 can be used in different ways, as a sauce for pasta, or as a topping for a baked potato. Ring the changes!

More substantial snacks include home-made pizzas – the children could help make these – cheese on toast (my fancy version is still much appreciated), small pasties and nutritious muffins. Some of these can be put in a packed lunch or, if in a small enough quantity, for eating at break time (although I'm much more in favour of fruit, now the norm in most schools for Key Stage 1 children). Some of the biscuits/cakes in the last chapter could be eaten at break time as well.

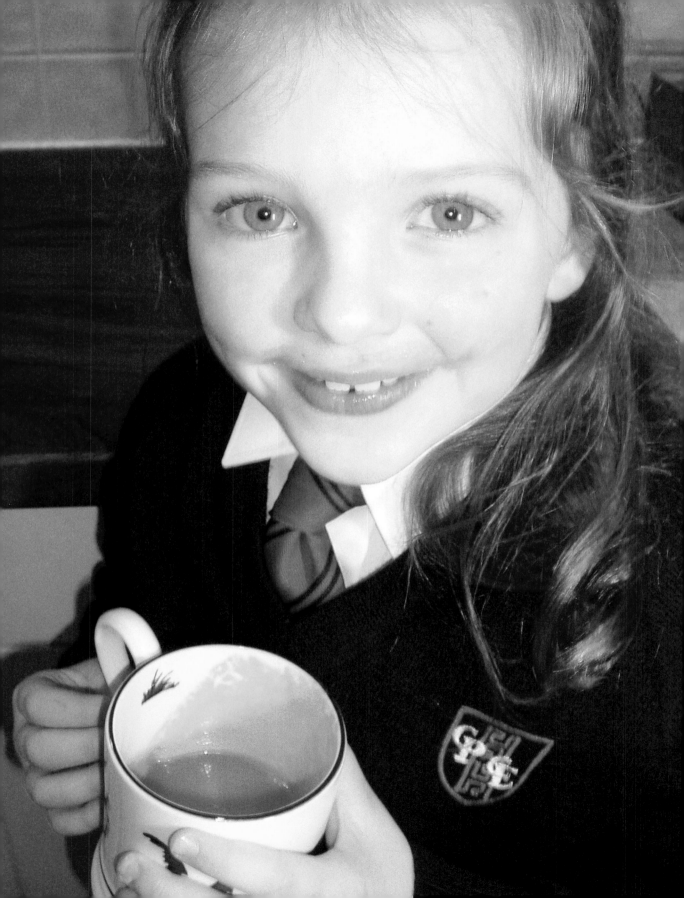

Soups

Basic stock

You can use this stock as the basis for any of the following soups, or in gravies. If making a poultry stock, use chicken, duck, turkey – or game bones if you have them. You can use cooked bones, left after you have eaten a bird or roast, but raw bones make a stronger-tasting stock. For a vegetable stock, omit the meat bones, double the quantity of vegetables, and add a leek and a couple of garlic cloves, with a slice or two of lemon as well if you like.

MAKES ABOUT 1.2 LITRES (2 pints)

1 bird carcass or some meat bones (lamb, beef or ham), broken up
1.5 litres (2¾ pints) water
1 large onion, peeled and halved
2 carrots, quartered
2 celery sticks, chopped
6 black peppercorns
2 bay leaves and a sprig of fresh thyme or rosemary
   (or a bouquet garni)

Freeze in handy pots, well labelled.

● Place all the ingredients in a large saucepan, and bring to the boil. Skim off any scum, and then reduce the heat, and put the lid on. Leave the poultry or meat stock to simmer for about 3 hours, skimming occasionally. Simmer the vegetable stock for about 30 minutes only.

● Cool slightly, then strain through a colander into a large bowl. When cool, strain through a fine sieve. May be kept in the fridge for up to 2 days.

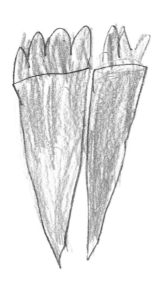

Basic cream of vegetable soup

If you follow the basic method below, and chop and change, using some of the vegetable ideas, you will be able to serve healthy and satisfying soups that no-one will ever tire of. Soups, of course, are never on the menu at school – for health and safety reasons – but at home a soup, accompanied by some crusty bread, can be a great snack after school, or the basis of a lunch or supper.

I've given quantities here for making more than four servings: you might as well make more while you are at it as these soups freeze well. The quantities given are based on prepared vegetables. You can make a soup simply from one vegetable or from a mixture. You can also have fun garnishing the soup (see page 227).

FOR 6–8 SMALL PORTIONS

55g (2oz) unsalted butter
175g (6oz) onions, finely chopped
400g (14oz) prepared vegetables, chopped into similar-sized pieces
    (see below for combinations)
1.2 litres (2 pints) stock (see page 223)
salt and pepper

Allow soup to cool, then pour into a freezerproof container.

● Melt the butter in a large soup pan, and fry the onions very gently until softened, about 20 minutes – don't let them brown. Add the prepared vegetable pieces, and stir around to coat them in butter. Add about 150ml (5fl oz) water or stock (when cooking for special occasions, you could use dry sherry or white wine instead), and cover the pot. Leave on a very, very low heat for about 30 minutes, stirring from time to time to make sure the liquid hasn't evaporated. The vegetables will be very soft.

● Add the cold stock to the pan, and then liquidize the soup in batches. As each batch is done, pour it into a sieve set over a clean saucepan. Press through with a pestle or the back of your soup ladle.

● When all the soup has been sieved, reheat very gently, and then add pepper to taste. In some of the individual recipes, you might want to add some different flavourings at this stage. For instance, add curry powder to the onion base, and you have an instant curried vegetable soup!

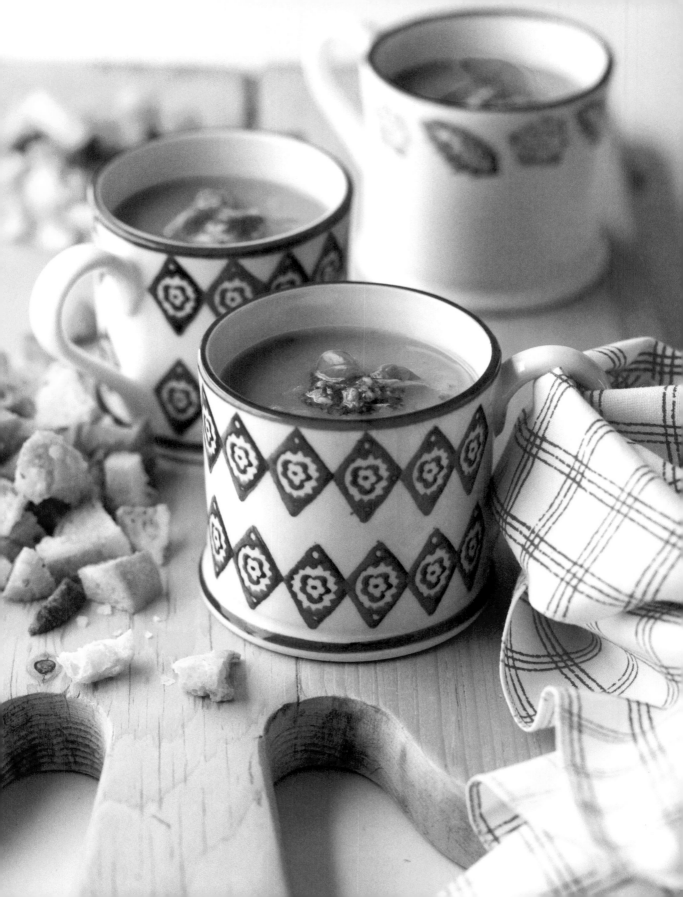

Soup variations

Broccoli and Apple Soup Use 200g (7oz) each of broccoli and apples – a sharp variety of the latter is more interesting. You can cook the apples, skin, core and all, as you will be sieving the end result.

Carrot and Apple Soup Use 250g (9oz) carrots and 150g (5oz) sharp apples. Again, you don't need to peel or core the apples or carrots, although most carrots are better peeled before you weigh them.

Carrot and Leek Soup Use 200g (7oz) each of carrots and leeks, having washed the latter very carefully, and trimmed off the ends and the toughest green of the leaves.

Carrot and Orange Soup Use 400g (14oz) carrots, and add the finely grated rind of 3 oranges when cooking the carrots. Add the juice of the oranges when liquidizing.

Cauliflower Cheese Soup Use 400g (14oz) cauliflower florets, and perhaps a few tiny ones for a garnish. Add a teaspoon each of freshly grated nutmeg and dry mustard powder to the onions with the cauliflower. Sprinkle each portion with very finely grated Cheddar when serving.

Leek and Potato Soup Use 200g (7oz) each of well-washed and trimmed leeks and peeled potatoes.

Mushroom and Apple Soup The tanginess of the apple will 'disguise' the mushrooms, for those who don't like the latter. Use 200g (7oz) each of sharp apples and fresh mushrooms – button or half-open ones are best – and don't forget to add the mushroom stalks as well, as they hold a lot of flavour.

Curried Parsnip Soup Use 400g (14oz) peeled parsnips, adding 2 teaspoons mild curry powder.

Pea and Sweetcorn Soup Use 200g (7oz) each of frozen peas and sweetcorn, and cook for only 10 minutes. To give extra flavour, add some lemon juice, or even some lemon pieces, which you liquidize along with the vegetables.

Pea and Mint Soup Use 400g (14oz) frozen peas, and about 4–6 sprigs fresh mint. Cook for 5–10 minutes only with the onions. Garnish with fresh mint and some extra peas. Some lemon juice could be added.

Pumpkin Soup Use 400g (14oz) flesh, skinned and seeded, of a very ripe pumpkin or squash.

Pumpkin and Apple Soup Use 200g (7oz) each of ripe pumpkin or squash and tart apples.

Spinach and Apple Soup Use 250g (9oz) defrosted frozen spinach (or that weight of cooked and squeezed fresh spinach) and 140g (5oz) sharp apples. A little freshly grated nutmeg is a good flavouring to add to the onions.

Squash, Sweet Potato and Swede Soup Use 130g (a generous 4½oz) of each ingredient.

Tomato Soup I think you must have the hang of it by now! Use 400g (14oz) tomatoes, preferably plum, which you should quarter first. You don't need to seed them, as you are going to sieve the soup after cooking.

Tomato and Apple Soup Use 200g (7oz) each of tomatoes and sharp apples.

Tomato, Celery and Apple Soup Use 130g (a generous 4½oz) of each ingredient.

Watercress and Potato Soup Use 100g (3½oz) peeled potatoes, which you cook for the 30 minutes. Add 300g (10½oz) washed watercress for the last 5 minutes, then liquidize. Add a little milk or cream at the end.

Soup garnishes

Often a soup will have an obvious garnish – a few peas or a mint leaf for a pea and mint soup, for instance – but here are a few general ideas that can enhance the taste, look and texture of a soup.

Croûtons Cut the crusts off day-old slices of bread, and cut the bread into small squares. Dry these in a low oven. You could also fry them or bake them in a little butter and oil. You could cut croûtons bigger, and put some grated cheese on them; if you grill them as you would cheese on toast, they're a delicious accompaniment to some soups.

Herbs These are an obvious garnish. Chop some leaves finely – parsley, coriander, sage – or leave them whole or in sprigs.

Bacon Cut rinded bacon rashers into tiny pieces, and fry or bake until crisp. Or simply cook the rashers whole until crisp then cut, chop or crush into pieces.

Vegetables or fruit Use tiny pieces of the soup's main fruit or vegetable raw on top of the soup when serving – tiny florets of broccoli or cauliflower, some apple dice, a broad bean, a sliver of celery or radish, peas or sweetcorn.

Nuts and seeds Toasted nuts or seeds are good on soups. Try pumpkin or sunflower seeds, or slivered almonds, pine kernels or sliced hazelnuts.

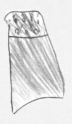

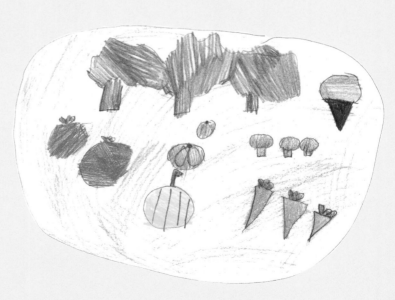

Dips and spreads

Avocado and tomato dip

This is a well-known Mexican dip – guacamole – made with the avocados that grow everywhere. It can be made much hotter, using a seeded and very finely chopped chilli, but this one is quite gentle. For an even creamier effect, add some cream cheese – about 115g (4oz) – or 2–3 tablespoons low-fat mayonnaise. Serve with crudités (sticks of raw veg), toast, pitta bread, breadsticks (see page 246), in sandwiches or on tortillas.

SERVES 4

1 large avocado
juice of 1 lime (or lemon)
1 large tomato, very finely diced (skinned if you like)
1 tablespoon finely chopped onion or spring onion
2 tablespoons crème fraîche or fromage frais
2 tablespoons chopped fresh coriander

● Cut open the avocados and remove the stones. Peel and chop the flesh into a bowl. Mash with a fork, adding the lime juice as you do so. Add the tomato, onion, crème fraîche or fromage frais and coriander to the avocado. Mix well, and season to taste.

● Serve with tortilla chips. (To make a healthier version at home, buy flat tortillas, cut them into triangles, brush with olive oil, and bake for a few minutes in a moderate oven until crisp.)

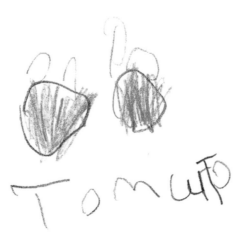

Tomuto

Sun-dried tomato salsa

Serve with fingers of raw vegetables, toast, pitta bread, breadsticks (see page 246) or potato wedges. Good with some plain fish as well.

SERVES 4

1 tomato, deseeded and finely chopped
25g (1oz) sun-dried tomatoes, finely chopped
25g (1oz) capers, rinsed and chopped
1 tablespoon olive oil
1 red chilli, seeded and finely chopped (optional)

● Combine all the ingredients in a bowl and mix well.

Mango salsa

Salsa is actually the Spanish for sauce, and this dip can be used as a sauce (it would be good with a plain baked piece of fish). Serve with tortilla chips, breadsticks (see page 246) or pitta bread. Be very careful not to touch your eyes after handling the chilli.

SERVES 4

600g (1lb 5oz) ripe mangoes
1 small green chilli, deseeded and finely chopped (optional)
6 spring onions, trimmed and finely chopped
225g (8oz) medium tomatoes, deseeded and finely chopped
2–3 tablespoons chopped fresh coriander
3 tablespoons olive oil
1 tablespoon lemon juice

● Peel the mango. Cut on either side of the large central flat stone and slice the flesh away from the stone. Chop the flesh into tiny cubes, and put in a bowl.

● Add all of the remaining ingredients to the mango and mix well.

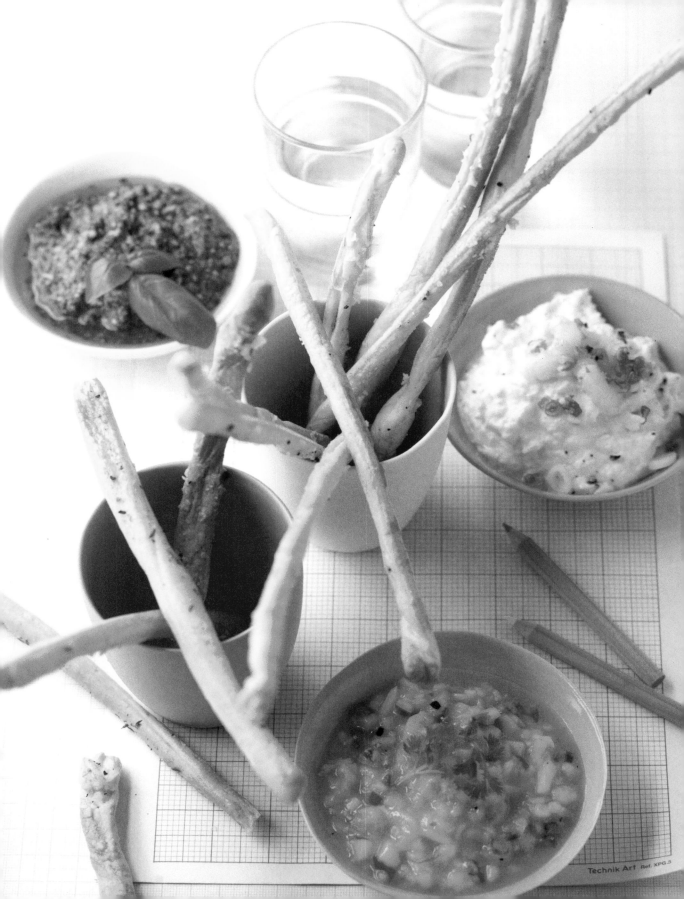

Pineapple and mango salsa

This is good as an accompaniment for grilled meats, poultry or grilled shellfish – particularly the Chicken Maryland on page 152. Children love the sweetness!

SERVES 4

140g (5oz) pineapple flesh, finely chopped
1 small ripe mango, peeled, stoned and finely chopped
1 large ripe tomato, deseeded and finely chopped
2 spring onions, finely chopped
1 tablespoon tomato ketchup
1 tablespoon olive oil

● Mix all the ingredients together in a bowl.

Basil or parsley pesto

Pesto is a great sauce made from Parmesan cheese, basil and pine kernels, which is mainly used on pasta. But a pesto can be made from other herbs, or even from vegetables (raw broccoli pesto is healthy and delicious). Parsley is widely available, and a pesto made from it can be used as a dip, spread or pasta sauce (try adding some to mashed potato!). You can use another Italian cheese, pecorino, instead of the Parmesan, and in some parts of Italy they use walnuts instead of the pine kernels.

SERVES 4

55g (2oz) Parmesan cheese, freshly grated
25g (1oz) pine kernels
1 large garlic clove, peeled and finely chopped
55g (2oz) fresh basil or parsley leaves
a squeeze of lemon juice
150ml (5fl oz) olive oil

● Put everything except for the oil in the food processor and blend until smooth. Add the oil gradually with the motor running.

● Serve as a dip. If using as a pasta sauce, dilute with a little more olive oil.

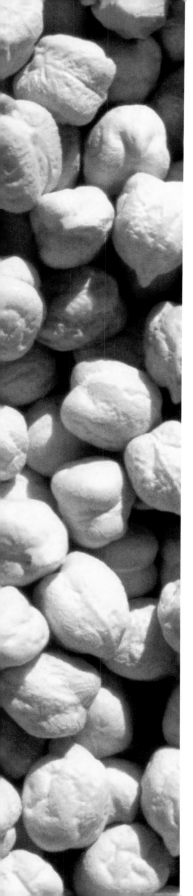

Ginger and prawn dip

Serve with vegetable sticks – courgette, radish, fennel, cucumber. You can use smoked trout or smoked salmon instead of prawns.

SERVES 4

140g (5oz) peeled prawns
85g (3oz) cream cheese
4 tablespoons crème fraîche
2 tablespoons lemon juice

½ teaspoon grated fresh
    root ginger
1 teaspoon chopped
    fresh chives

● If the prawns are large, remove the dark veins. Save 25g (1oz) of them for decoration.

● Put everything apart from the chives into the food processor and blend until smooth.

● Chill and serve with the chives and reserved prawns, whole or chopped, sprinkled on top.

Chickpea and herb dip

This is a variation on the Middle Eastern hummus.

SERVES 4

1 x 400g can chickpeas,
    rinsed and drained
2 tablespoons finely chopped
    fresh coriander or mint leaves
2 spring onions, finely chopped

1 garlic clove, peeled and
    finely chopped
juice of 1 lemon
8 tablespoons olive oil

● Put the chickpeas in the food processor with the herb, spring onion, garlic and lemon juice, and blend. Add the olive oil very slowly. Blend until smooth.

● Spoon into a bowl and serve.

Cucumber, yoghurt and mint dip

This is a variation on the Greek tzatziki, or the raita served in Indian restaurants. It is very cooling when eaten with a hot curry, but it is delicious on its own as a dip, and very good indeed as a topping for a baked potato.

SERVES 4

1 small cucumber, about 175g (6oz)
300ml (10fl oz) natural bio-live yoghurt
2 tablespoons finely chopped fresh mint
½ teaspoon ground cumin
freshly ground black pepper

● Peel the cucumber, and grate it into a bowl. Stir the yoghurt until creamy and smooth, then mix into the cucumber along with the mint, cumin and some pepper.

● If you like, sprinkle a little more cumin and/or pepper over the top. Chill before serving.

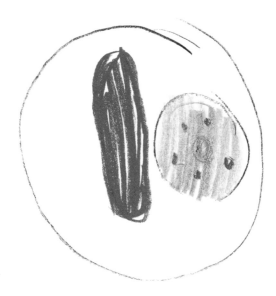

Tuna and olive dip

The Mediterranean flavours here – of tuna, olives and capers – might be a bit strong for some younger children, but you could be surprised. I have met many children who eat olives as enthusiastically as they might sweets! This can be used as a dip, or it can be spread on toast or lengths of celery, or stuffed into small hollowed-out tomatoes. This makes a great sandwich filling, and is delicious with baked potatoes. For a Provençal tapenade, add some anchovies.

SERVES 4

55g (2oz) pitted black olives
25g (1oz) bottled capers, drained and rinsed
1 small garlic clove, peeled and crushed
juice of ½ lemon
1 teaspoon dry mustard powder
3 tablespoons natural bio-live yoghurt, fromage frais or crème fraîche
55g (2oz) canned tuna in spring water, drained and flaked
2 tablespoons olive oil

● Put everything except the tuna and oil in the food processor and blend until smooth.

● Add the tuna, then pour in the oil in gradually, with the machine running, adding more if you want the texture to be runnier. Don't over-process the tuna, as it becomes very grainy.

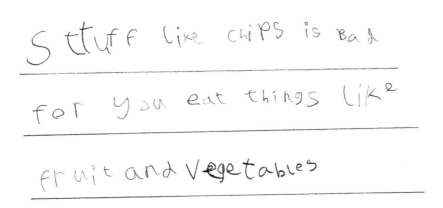

S ttuff like chiPs is Bad
for you eat things like
fruit and vegetables

Snacks

Tuna and cheese muffins

These make a change from sandwiches after school. They're also very good as a light lunch with some carrot and cucumber sticks and baby tomatoes.

SERVES 4

4 large spring onions, finely sliced
olive oil
175g(6oz) canned tuna in spring water
3 tablespoons low-fat mayonnaise
2 tablespoons sunflower seeds (optional)
4 brown or white muffins
115g (4oz) Edam cheese, grated

● Preheat the oven to 200°C/400°F/Gas 6.

● Fry the spring onion in a little olive oil until soft, about 5 minutes. Drain the tuna and flake into a mixing bowl. Add the onion, mayonnaise and sunflower seeds, if using. Mix well.

● Split and toast the muffins. Pile the tuna mixture on to the halved muffins and sprinkle the grated cheese on the top.

● Bake in the preheated oven for 10–15 minutes until the cheese is golden brown and bubbling. Serve hot.

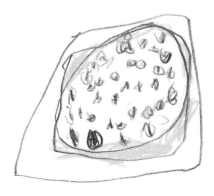

Fancy cheese on toast

This is a meal in itself, great when children are hungry and in a rush. There is nothing like the taste and smell of good fresh bread – for it's not called the staff of life for nothing. There is now a huge selection of breads around, some with olives and peppers added, or cheese and herbs. Ciabatta would be good.

SERVES 4

1 tablespoon olive oil
4 rashers bacon, rinded
4 slices bread, thickly cut
55g (2oz) pesto (see page 232)
55g (2oz) spinach leaves, washed
115g (4oz) Red Leicester cheese, grated

● Heat the olive oil in a small frying pan and cook the bacon for 5–10 minutes until crisp.

● Preheat the grill, and toast the bread on both sides. Spread the pesto evenly on the bread, making sure you go right to the edges of the bread.

● In a small saucepan bring a little water to the boil. Add the spinach and cook for 1 minute. Drain very well, and divide the spinach between the pieces of toast. Lay the bacon on top of the spinach, and sprinkle with the cheese.

● Cook under the preheated grill until bubbling and golden brown.

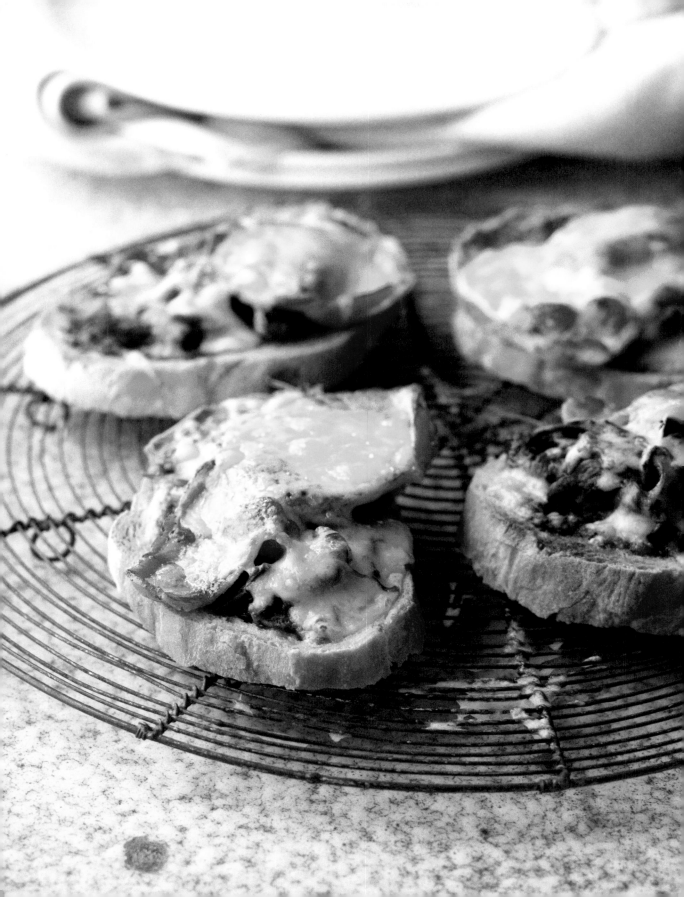

Pizzas

Pizza has developed from being the thrifty Italian housewife's way of using up leftovers on a baked bread base, to being a worldwide passion. There are chains of pizza restaurants now, and most of them are very good – it's a form of fast food that is not too unhealthy – but the ones you make at home are much tastier, and you can vary the toppings almost indefinitely. I give a recipe for a basic pizza dough here, but you could also use many other types of base (see opposite). I think children like pizza because it can be eaten in their hands.

MAKES 2 x 25cm (10in) pizza bases

250g (9oz) strong white flour
1½ teaspoons fast-acting dried yeast
50ml (2fl oz) olive oil, plus extra for greasing
50ml (2fl oz) lukewarm water

● Sift the flour into a large bowl along with the yeast, and make a well in the centre. Add the oil and the water, and mix with a wooden spoon, adding a little more water if necessary, until you have a soft dough.

● Turn out on to a floured work surface and knead energetically for about 10 minutes until the dough is soft and has a shine to it. Put it into a lightly oiled bowl, turn around to coat with oil, then cover with a tea-towel. Leave in a warm place for about 1½ hours, or until the dough has doubled in size.

● Preheat the oven to 200°C/400°F/Gas 6.

● Turn the dough out on to a lightly floured surface and puncture it – it's known as 'knocking it back' – with your knuckles. Knead for a few more minutes, then divide the dough in half. Roll each piece of dough out to a 25cm (10in) circle – or you could try easing the dough out into a circle with the heel of your hand. Leave the edges slightly thicker, to prevent the topping running off. Place on a couple of lightly oiled baking sheets.

● Top the pizza bases with the topping of your choice (see opposite). Bake in the preheated oven for 15–20 minutes, or until the top is sizzling and the crusts are golden.

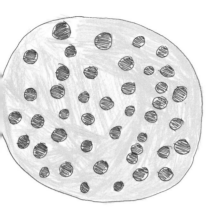

Pizza toppings

Napoletana (plain tomato) Spread the pizza base with some thick tomato sauce made with garlic (see page 142), and sprinkle it with some dried oregano and olive oil.

Margherita (tomato, mozzarella and basil) Spread the base with tomato sauce as above, then top with slices of mozzarella (best from little 150g packets in brine). Sprinkle with torn basil leaves and olive oil.

Due Formaggi (two cheeses) The classic pizza-chain cheese pizza uses four cheeses – and of course you can do this. Use about 115g (4oz) of each cheese if going for the two-cheese option, 55g (2oz) of each if using four cheeses. Mozzarella and Cheddar are good, and you could add a final sprinkling of Parmesan. Drizzle with olive oil before baking.

Bacon and cheese Fry some little strips of thickish bacon rashers or Italian bacon (pancetta) and place on top of the pizza base, with or without tomato sauce. Place slices of mozzarella on top, and drizzle with olive oil.

Other pizza topping ingredients
The essence of ingredients for pizza topping is that they are small enough to cook quickly, in the 15–20 minutes or so of baking. Some ideas . . .

- Strips of green or red pepper
- Slices of tomato
- Anchovy fillets
- Slices of chorizo, pepperoni or other spicy sausage
- Black or green olives, stoned
- Blanched slices of fennel
- Sliced mushrooms
- Canned tuna (look for the tuna canned in spring water)
- Capers
- A pinch of chilli flakes in the tomato sauce, for heat . . .
- A sprinkling of a soft herb, like dried oregano or fresh basil or thyme

Alternative pizza bases You can use anything you like. A pizza base, after all, is only a thin layer of bread, so you can use toasted sliced bread at its simplest. But you can also use other types of bread: halved toasted bap rolls, crumpets, or baguettes. Cut the baguette into four pieces, then split each piece in half. Top with tomato sauce, cheese and anything else you fancy, then drizzle with a little olive oil. Place under the grill until the cheese is beginning to brown.

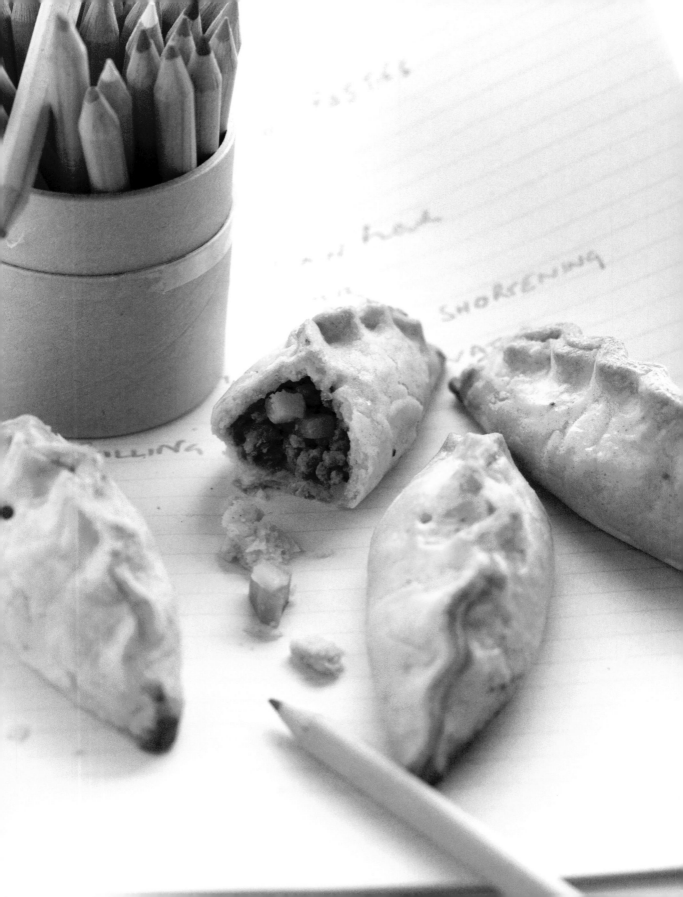

Cornish pasties

Cornish pasties are usually huge, and can out-face a small child (as well as an adult!), so I have made these smaller than they usually are. They are delicious, even though I say so myself.

MAKES 4

For the pastry
225g (8oz) plain flour
55g (2oz) butter, diced
55g (2oz) vegetable shortening, diced
2 tablespoons water

For the filling
225g (8oz) minced lamb
1 teaspoon Worcestershire sauce

115g (4oz) swede, peeled and finely chopped
115g (4oz) carrot, peeled and finely chopped
115g (4oz) onions, peeled and finely chopped
1 tablespoon plain flour, mixed with 250ml (9fl oz) water until smooth
15g (½oz) Marmite

These freeze very well before or after cooking.

● Make the pastry as described on page 66. Wrap in clingfilm and place in the fridge.

● To prepare the filling, put the meat in a saucepan with about 50ml (2fl oz) water and the Worcestershire sauce, and simmer for 10 minutes. Add the vegetables, flour and water, and Marmite, and continue to cook, stirring, for about 5–10 minutes until the sauce has thickened. Remove from the heat and leave to cool.

● Preheat the oven to 200°C/400°F/Gas 6.

● Take the pastry out of the fridge, bring it to room temperature and divide into four pieces. Roll each piece out into a circle, or use a saucer of about 15cm (6in) diameter and cut around it. Dampen the edges with water. Divide the lamb and vegetable mixture between the four circles, fold over and pinch the edges together like a pleat.

● Put the pasties on a baking tray and bake in the preheated oven for 10 minutes, then reduce the heat to 180°C/350°F/Gas 4. Bake for a further 20–25 minutes until the pasties are golden brown and cooked through.

Cheese twists

These are great as a quick snack, or to use with a dip, or you could have them when the children aren't around, with drinks. You could use any cheese, but Parmesan is very good. You can also add other flavours: try adding a teaspoon of garlic salt, or some anchovy fillets (soaked in milk first).

MAKES ABOUT 20

115g (4oz) self-raising flour
a pinch of English mustard powder
55g (2oz) unsalted butter, cut into small cubes
85g (3oz) strong cheese, grated
1 teaspoon chopped fresh chives
1 egg, beaten

❄
Freeze when baked, packed into a freezerproof container.

● Preheat the oven to 180°C/350°F/Gas 4.

● Sieve the flour and mustard into the processor with the butter, and process until the mixture is like breadcrumbs. Add the cheese, chopped chives and egg, and blend in quick bursts until it comes together to form a dough.

● Roll out on a lightly floured board very thinly. Cut into strips of about 18cm (7in) long and 1cm (½in) wide. Twist and place on a baking tray. Bake in the preheated oven for 10–15 minutes. When cool, store in an airtight container.

Melba toast

I remember this used to be very popular about twenty years ago, served in restaurants with pâté. It deserves to be brought back into favour, though, as it is crisp, tasty and good with creamy dips (see pages 229–35). Melba toast can be made a few days in advance, if kept in an airtight container.

MAKES 16–32 PIECES

4 slices brown or granary bread (sliced is best)

● Preheat the oven to 180°C/350°F/Gas 4.

● Toast the bread slices on both sides. Cut off the crusts. Slice each piece of toast through the middle, horizontally, to make two thin slices. Cut these slices in half diagonally into triangles (and then in half again diagonally if you like, to make even smaller triangles).

● Arrange the 'toasts' on a baking sheet and bake in the preheated oven for about 10 minutes until golden and crisp and beginning to curl up at the edges. Watch them carefully as they can burn very quickly.

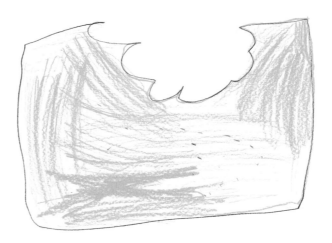

Breadsticks

Known as 'grissini' in Italy, these crisp sticks made from a basic bread dough can be served with a first course or dip – or just as a snack. You can vary them by adding white or black sesame seeds to the dough – or sprinkling them on afterwards – or sprinkle with coarse salt, grated Parmesan cheese, fresh thyme or rosemary leaves. Children enjoy making, shaping and decorating these. They will keep for up to a week in an airtight tin.

MAKES ABOUT 20 STICKS

1 teaspoon dried yeast
125ml (4fl oz) lukewarm water
225g (8oz) strong plain flour
about 2½ tablespoons olive oil
1 tablespoon poppyseeds (optional)
1–2 tablespoons cornmeal or semolina
1 egg yolk, mixed with a little water

❆

After freezing and defrosting, refresh in a warm oven until crisp again.

● Whisk the yeast and water together in a small bowl, and leave to dissolve for about 5 minutes.

● Put the flour in a large bowl and make a well in the centre. Pour in the yeast liquid and olive oil, and gradually mix together to a dough. Add poppy seeds now if desired. Turn on to a lightly floured work surface and knead until smooth. Place in a lightly floured bowl, cover and leave to rise in a warm place until doubled in size, about 40–60 minutes.

● Knead the dough again, then shape into a rectangle of about 30 x 20cm (12 x 8in). Cover and rest again for 10 minutes.

● Preheat the oven to 200°C/400°F/Gas 6.

● Cut the rectangle of dough in half across the width, and then cut each smaller rectangle into 10 pieces lengthways. Roll and stretch each of these to about 25cm (10in) long.

● Dust two baking sheets with the cornmeal or semolina, and arrange the dough sticks on them, spaced well apart. Brush with the egg glaze and sprinkle with seeds now if you want (if you haven't put them in the dough). Bake in the preheated oven for about 10–15 minutes until golden and crisp. Cool on a wire rack.

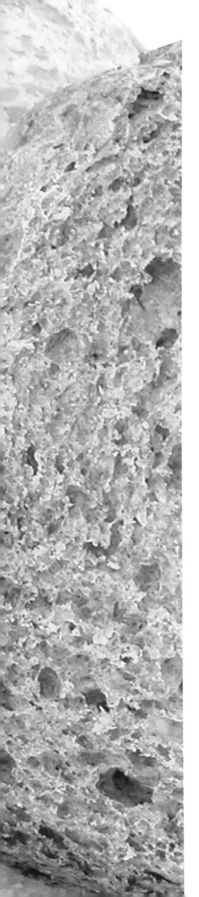

All sorts of sandwiches ▶

There are so many varieties of bread nowadays, and artisan bakers seem to be making a comeback. I think it is worth buying good organic brown bread, but you can try bagels, or bread with sun-dried tomatoes, olives, pumpkin seeds or mixed seeds. You could also try pitta bread pockets and tortilla wraps.

Simply slice the bread as thick as you like (but not too thick), and fill generously. Perhaps one slice could be white, one brown. You could make pinwheel sandwiches for a change. Just cover one slice with filling, then roll up the bread, wrap in clingfilm and leave in the fridge to 'set'. Take off the clingfilm, slice into little round pinwheels, and serve. The children can help make these when they come in from school shouting 'I'm starving.'

Filling suggestions

- Tuna and sweetcorn with a little mayonnaise

- Ham and cream cheese

- Roasted tomatoes and sausage (cook the sausage the night before)

- Cheese and mango chutney

- Tuna and carrot (shred the carrot finely)

- Cream cheese and finely sliced pitted olives mixed together (use olives sparingly so the children get used to the taste)

- Bacon and egg (cook the bacon and boil the egg the night before, then chop up into small pieces)

The list is endless so let your imagination – and the children's – go free!

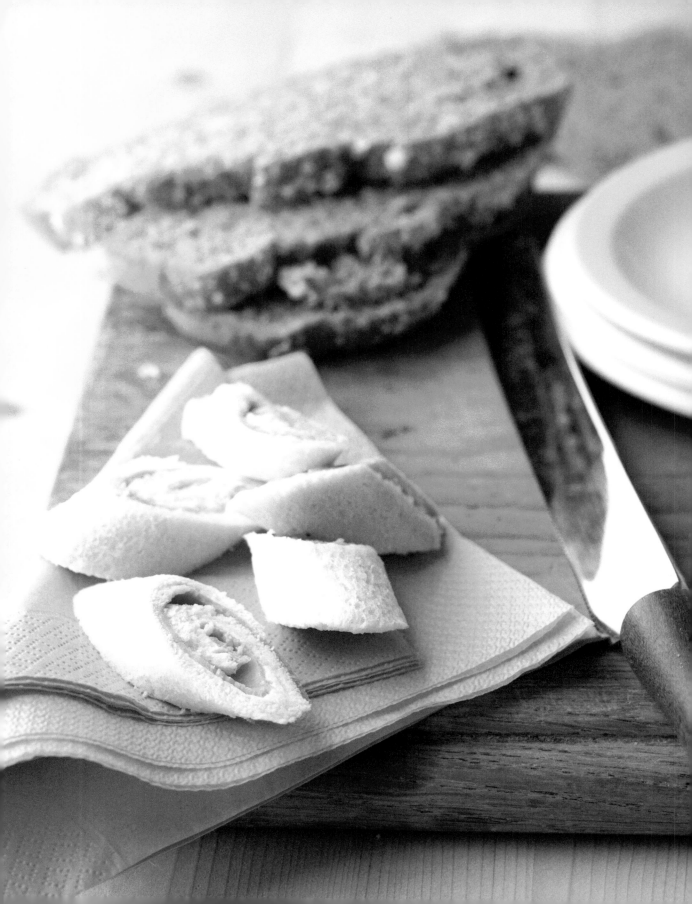

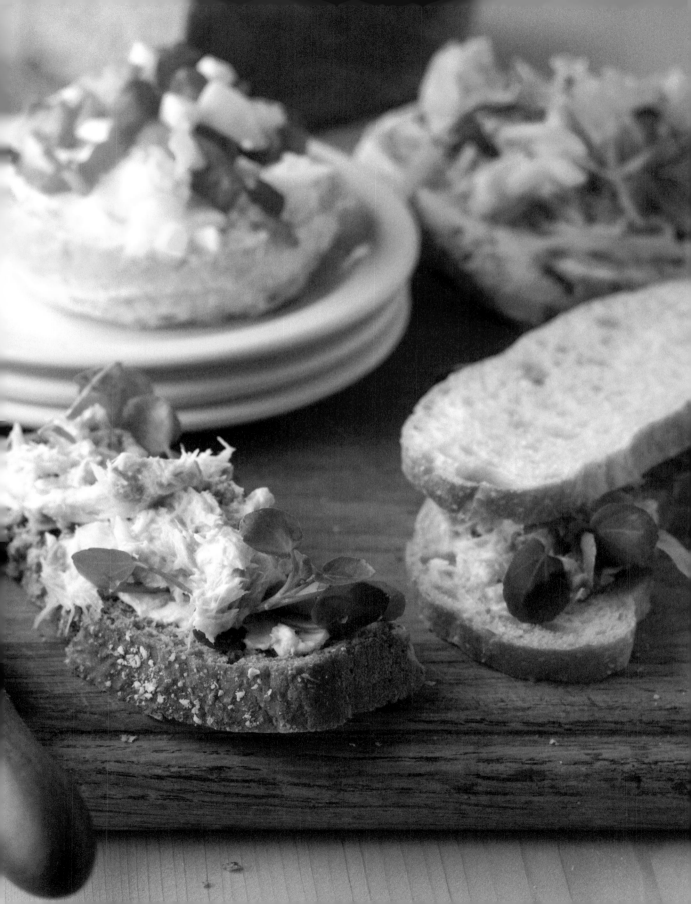

Sweet things

Children love sweet things. I know sugar is frowned upon, but if you make your own desserts, cakes and biscuits, at least you know how *much* sugar (and what kind) you have used. This way you can offer them something home-made as a treat every now and again.

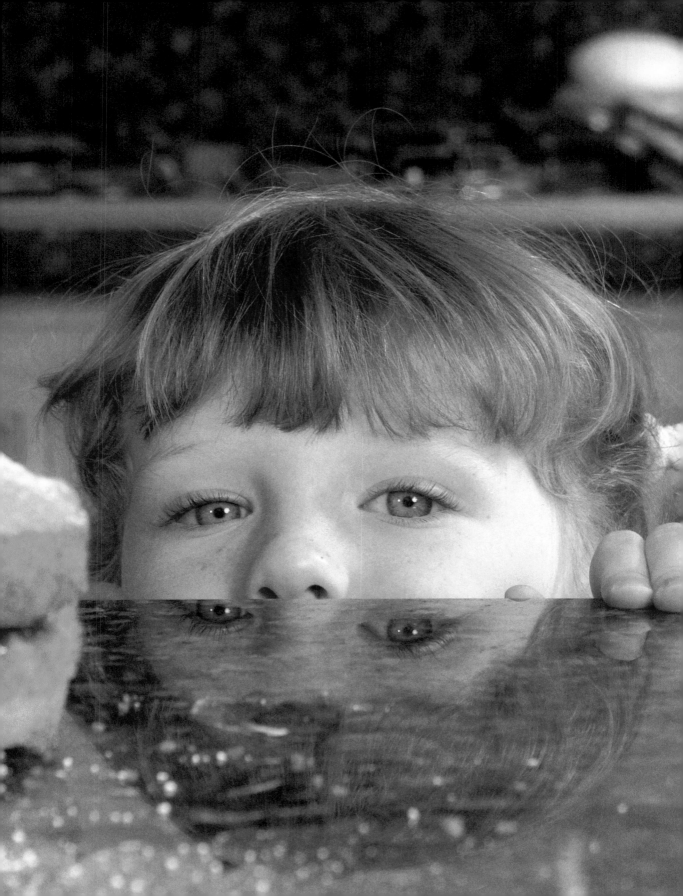

FRUIT IS THE MOST nutritious sweet food, and this would be my first choice to serve after a main course or a bowl of soup, or just as a snack. Remember that young children can be 'outfaced' by a large apple or pear, and will be more likely to eat it if it's cut into smaller pieces. Fruit can be cooked in puddings and desserts too. I have included quite a few fruit recipes here, some of which are also suitable for breakfasts. Have a look too at the breakfast chapter for recipes that could be served as puddings.

Fruits, usually the soft variety, can be made into healthy sauces for puddings, fresh or cooked fruit, ice-creams or cake-type desserts. I've also given you a custard recipe which, flavoured with chocolate, is strictly for special occasions …

Biscuits and cakes can be time-consuming to make, I know, but if you batch-bake (see page 69), then store or freeze them, you will always have something ready for tea at the weekend, or for when the children come home from school. And the children can always help you make them too.

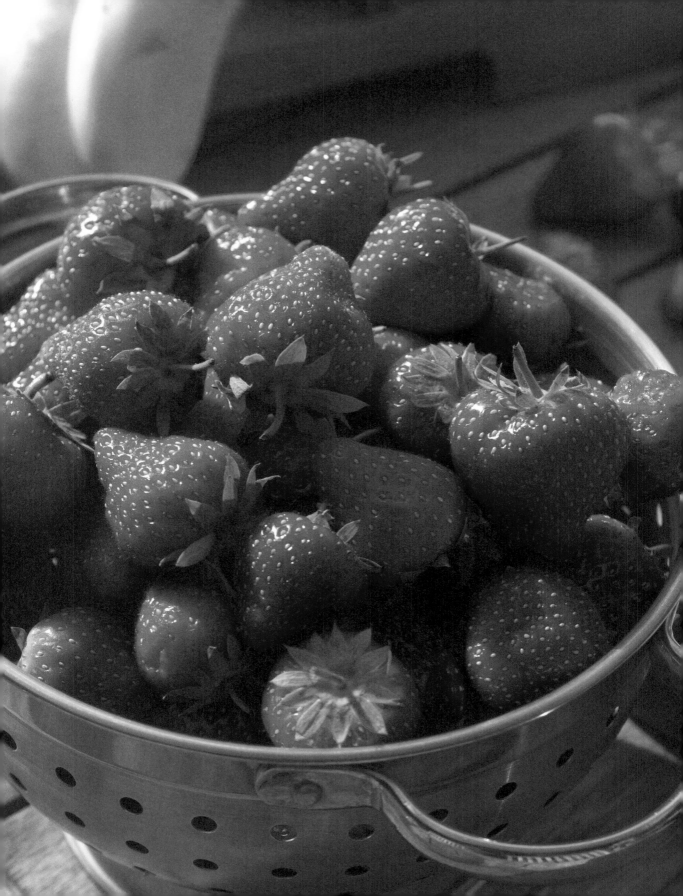

puddings

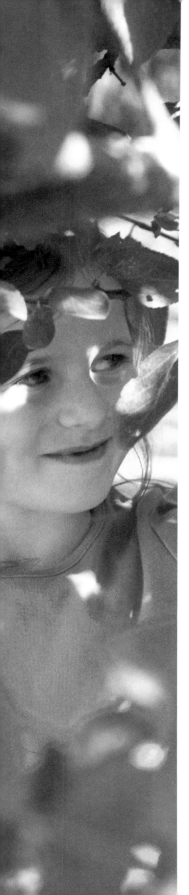

Apple whirligig

This recipe is from Margaret Patterson, the school cook at Hurlford Primary School in Ayrshire, Scotland. It was given to me after I visited the school as a judge for the Soil Association School Food Award. They won!

Margaret says you could ring the changes and seasons with this pudding, substituting gooseberries, plums or rhubarb for the apples. Always use a dark jam, though.

SERVES 4

55g (2oz) butter, diced, plus extra for greasing
450g (1lb) cooking apples, peeled, cored and sliced
2 tablespoons water
4 rounded tablespoons red jam
115g (4oz) self-raising flour
1 level tablespoon caster sugar
3 tablespoons semi-skimmed milk

● Preheat the oven to 220°C/425°F/Gas 7, and butter a shallow ovenproof dish.

● Place the apple slices in the dish. Blend the water with 2 tablespoons of the jam and pour over the apples. Bake in the preheated oven for 5–10 minutes until the apples are soft.

● Meanwhile, put the flour in a bowl with the sugar. Add the diced butter, and rub into the flour until the mixture resembles fine breadcrumbs. Add the milk and mix with a knife to make a firm dough.

● Roll the dough out on a floured board to an oblong 20 x 15cm (8 x 6in). Spread with the remaining jam, then roll up like a Swiss roll and cut into eight slices.

● Place the slices of dough around the edge of the apple dish, leaving a space between each. Return to the oven and bake for a further 15 minutes until the apples are tender and the 'scones' have risen and turned golden brown.

● Serve hot with real custard (see page 269).

Baked stuffed peaches

Peaches are delicious eaten whole in the hand like an apple – or stoned and in wedges for younger children. But they can also be baked, with a tasty filling in the hole left by the stone (macaroons contain nuts, so not for those with allergies). Nectarines can be cooked in the same way.

SERVES 4

4 large ripe peaches
55g (2oz) small macaroon biscuits (or sponge fingers), crushed
25g (1oz) ground almonds
300ml (10fl oz) apple juice
1 heaped tablespoon soft brown sugar

● Preheat the oven to 180°C/350°F/Gas 4.

● Cut the peaches in half, following the line around the fruit, and remove the stones. Carve the middles out a bit to make the holes larger. Keep the flesh, and chop it finely.

● Mix the chopped peach flesh with the biscuit crumbs, ground almonds and 50ml (2fl oz) of the apple juice. Fill the holes in the peaches with the mixture, and put the peaches in a baking dish, stuffing side up. Pour the rest of the apple juice around the peaches, and sprinkle the sugar over the tops of the peaches.

● Cover with a piece of foil and bake in the preheated oven for 20 minutes. Remove the foil and cook for a further 20 minutes.

● Allow to cool, then serve with the juices.

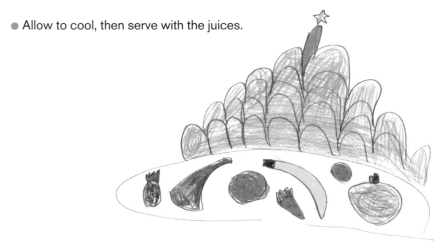

Fruit on a stick

Children enjoy these kebabs, and it is an easy way to increase their daily fruit intake. You will need some wooden skewers, which you should soak for a while before use to prevent splinters and burning.

SERVES 4

350g (12oz) pineapple, peeled, cored and cut into slices
115g (4oz) strawberries, washed and hulled
1 large banana
25g (1oz) soft dark brown sugar
1 tablespoon runny honey

● Preheat the grill.

● Cut the circles of pineapple flesh into 5cm (2in) chunks. Cut the hulled strawberries in half crossways. Peel the banana and cut into chunks the same size as the pineapple.

● Put the sugar and honey in a small saucepan and just warm through. Do not boil.

● Thread the fruit on to the skewers and brush with the honey mixture on all sides. Grill for 5 minutes or until lightly browned.

For a larger quantity

Prepare up to the stage of threading on to the skewers. Put the fruit in shallow baking trays and pour over the honey mixture. Stir well until coated, then bake in an oven preheated to 220°C/425°F/Gas 7 for 10 minutes or until lightly golden.

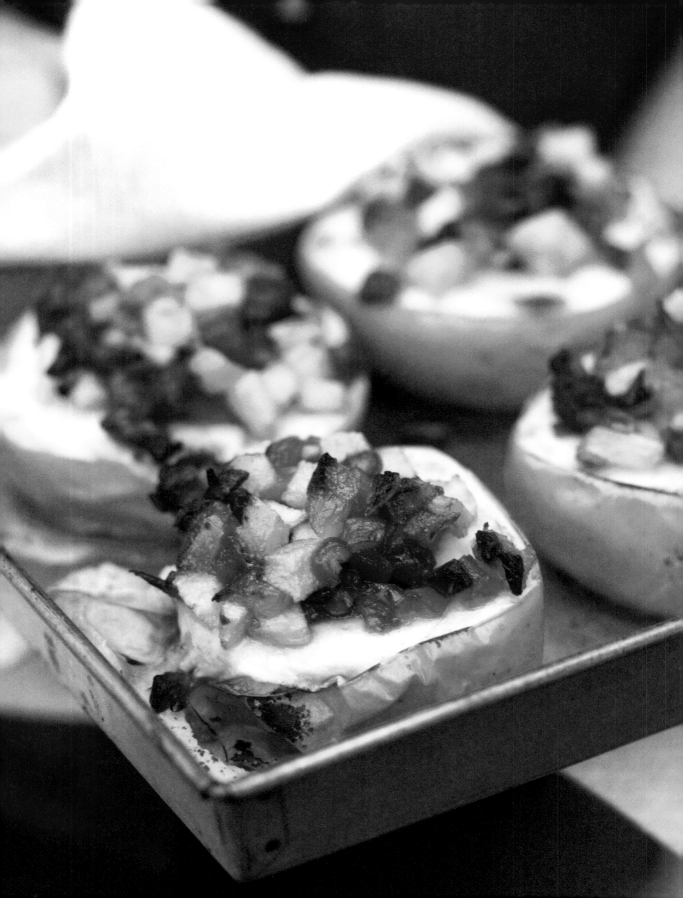

Baked apples

Great on a cold winter's night with lashings of real custard (see page 269). Use any mixture of dried or fresh fruit for the filling. But try my idea: the combination of pear and orange is quite special!

The apples can be assembled up to 2 hours in advance of the cooking. Put a little lemon juice over the cut sides of the apples to prevent them turning brown.

SERVES 4

4 medium cooking apples

For the filling
1 medium pear, peeled, cored and diced
55g (2oz) dried apricots, pre-soaked and diced
55g (2oz) stoned dates, diced
25g (1oz) sultanas
25g (1oz) demerara sugar
2 tablespoons orange juice

● Preheat the oven to 180°C/350°F/Gas 4.

● Combine the pear, apricots, dates and sultanas in a large bowl. Add the sugar and orange juice and stir well. Leave for about 20 minutes so that the fruit can soak up the orange juice.

● Wipe the apples with a cloth and take out the cores using an apple corer. Cut the apples in half through the middle, and place on a baking sheet, flat side up. Drain the fruit mixture and divide between the cavities in the apples with your fingers. Press the fruit down into the apple.

● Cover the baking sheet loosely with foil and bake in the preheated oven for 25–30 minutes until the apple is just soft.

● Serve with fresh custard or some natural bio-live yoghurt.

Poached pears

This is a delicious way of cooking pears. It's best to use ripe pears, but it works well for those hard ones you occasionally buy. The pears will keep in their syrup in the fridge for up to a week. Serve with some lemon sorbet.

SERVES 4

rind and juice of 1 lemon
1 cinnamon stick
½ teaspoon ground mixed spice
¼ teaspoon ground black pepper
600ml (1 pint) apple juice
4 ripe pears, peeled but with the stem left intact

● In a large saucepan, mix together the rind and lemon juice, cinnamon stick, spice, pepper, apple juice and 300ml (10fl oz) water.

● Hollow out the first 2.5cm (1in) of the core of each pear, and trim the base so they stand upright.

● Add the pears to the pan, and cover with a piece of parchment to prevent discolouring. Bring to the boil, then turn the heat down and simmer gently, without a lid, turning occasionally, for 20 minutes (depending on ripeness) or until tender at the base.

● Remove the pears from the pan and transfer to a bowl. Raise the heat and boil the liquid until reduced by half or until syrupy. Strain and leave to cool. Pour over the pears and refrigerate.

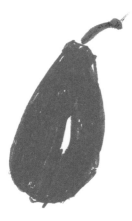

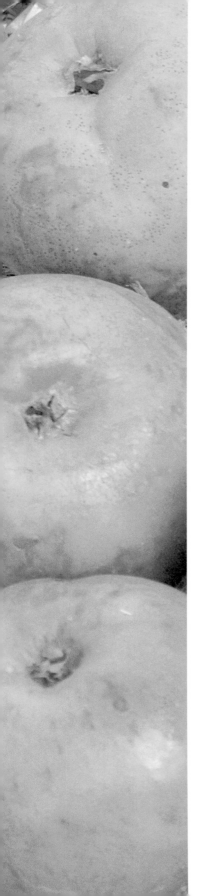

Stewed apples and blueberries

You could eat this by itself, and it is wonderful in a crumble, pie or pancake. Blueberries – also known as whortleberries or bilberries – are rich in Vitamin C and antioxidants (which protect against disease). A handful of blueberries provides as many antioxidants as five servings of carrots, apples or broccoli …

SERVES 4

675g (1½ lb) cooking apples, peeled, cored and sliced
225g (8oz) blueberries
150ml (5fl oz) water
85g (3oz) soft brown sugar

● Place the apple slices in a saucepan with the blueberries, water and sugar. Heat gently until the sugar melts, then bring to the boil. Turn off the heat.

● If you want to make this into a crumble or pie, do so now, and continue the cooking with the pie crust or crumble topping (bake in a 200°C/400°F/Gas 6 oven for 20 minutes).

● Serve hot or cold.

Fresh fruit jelly

If you don't want to use gelatine, use commercial jelly (follow the instructions). You can buy a vegetarian version of gelatine, or use agar-agar, made from seaweed (though it's difficult to find and quite complicated to use).

You could make this jelly with dried fruit. Follow the instructions for the dried fruit compote on page 113, adding some gelatine, and make the liquid up to the quantities as given in the recipe below. Don't use pineapple, however, as it contains an enzyme that prevents the gelatine setting.

SERVES 4

600g (1lb 5oz) fruit (a mixture of strawberries and raspberries, kiwi fruit and banana, or orange segments and melon, use your imagination!)
225ml (8fl oz) orange or apple juice
200ml (7fl oz) water
55g (2oz) caster sugar
2 x 11g sachets powdered gelatine (or 6 gelatine leaves softened in water, or agar-agar)
juice of 1 lime

● Hull, peel and trim the fruit as appropriate. Halve strawberries if they are large, slice kiwi fruit and bananas and cut melon into small chunks.

● Mix the juice and water together, and heat half of this in a small pan until it begins to simmer. Add the sugar and gelatine, and heat very gently until it dissolves completely. Do not boil. Add the remaining liquid and the lime juice, and leave to cool.

● Line a 900g (2lb) loaf tin with clingfilm (this makes it easier to turn out the finished jelly), and put in the fruit. You can simply mix it all together, or you could arrange it attractively. Remember that what you put on the bottom will be on the top when you turn the jelly out. Pour the cold jelly – before it begins to set – over the fruit, and leave to chill in the fridge until fully set.

● To turn out, dip the bottom of the tin in hot water (to loosen the base and sides), and invert on to a serving plate. Remove the clingfilm. Serve with natural bio-live yoghurt if you like.

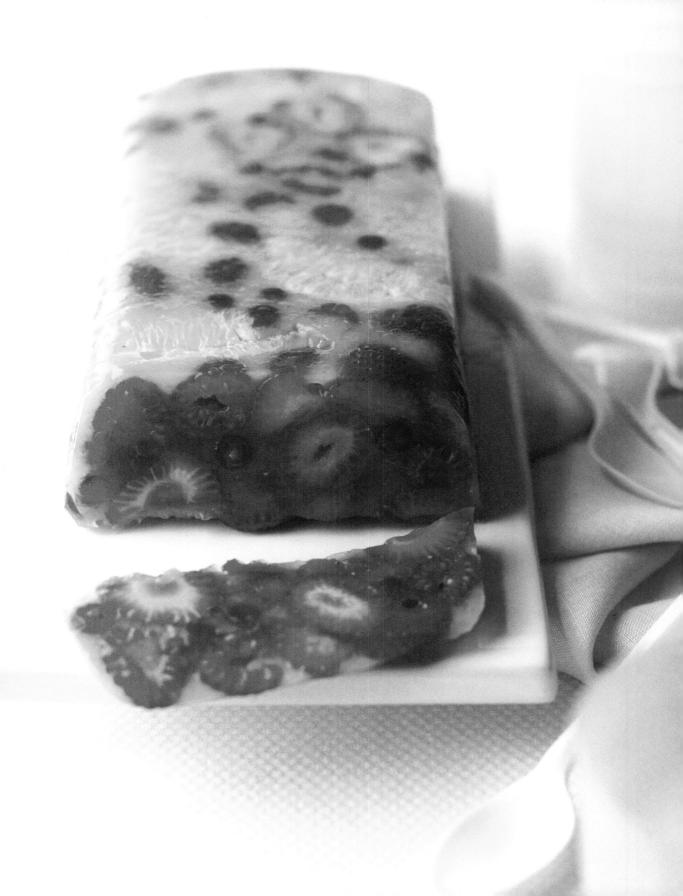

Summer pudding

This is a great favourite. You can either make one big one or, for a change, try making four small ones in teacups. The children love making these, and you could even take them to a fruit farm to pick the fruit first. Strawberries, raspberries, blackberries, blackcurrants, peaches and nectarines are all suitable in whatever proportions you prefer. If you are using peaches and nectarines, make sure they are really ripe: skin them and cut up very small (do this over a bowl so that you keep all the juice). Orange or raspberry juice can be used instead of the cranberry if you don't like the latter.

SERVES 4

450g (1lb) summer berries (see above)
25g (1oz) caster sugar
225g (8oz) white bread, crusts removed
200ml (7fl oz) cranberry juice

● Mix the berries together in a large bowl, add the sugar and mix again. Line a medium pudding basin with clingfilm, leaving an overhang.

● Cut a circle out of the bread for the bottom of the pudding basin, and cut the rest of the bread into fingers or shapes that will cover the sides. Put in a flat dish in one layer.

● Drain the juice from the fruit, and mix with the cranberry juice. Pour this over the bread to soak it. Line the pudding basin with most of the soaked bread – you will need some for the top of the bowl – and add the fruit. Put the remaining bread over the top of the pudding basin. Cover with clingfilm, and put a small plate with some weights on the top. Chill in the fridge for 2 hours until set.

● Remove the top clingfilm, and invert the pudding basin on to a plate. The pudding should slip out easily. Remove the remaining clingfilm. Serve with some crème fraîche or natural bio-live yoghurt.

Christmas pudding

The children at St Peter's really like this pudding, as it is quite light.
They can help with the mixing, but only one class per year, though!

SERVES 4

85g (3oz) apple, grated
85g (3oz) carrot, grated
½ lemon
½ orange
115g (4oz) currants
115g (4oz) mixed peel
115g (4oz) sultanas
55g (2oz) raisins
115g (4oz) self-raising flour

½ teaspoon freshly grated
  nutmeg
½ teaspoon mixed spice
115g (4oz) butter
115g (4oz) brown breadcrumbs
85g (3oz) brown sugar
1 egg
1 tablespoon golden syrup
1–2 tablespoons milk

● Combine the grated apple and carrot in a large bowl. Grate the rind of the lemon and orange into the bowl, and squeeze the juice in as well. Add all the dried fruit and mix well. Set to one side.

● In another large bowl mix the flour and spices together, then rub in the butter until the texture is like breadcrumbs. Add the actual breadcrumbs, then the dried-fruit mixture, the sugar, egg and syrup. Beat well, adding enough milk to give a dropping consistency. Don't forget to make a wish at this stage.

● Pour the mixture into a lightly oiled 1.2 litre (2 pint) pudding basin. Cut a circle of greaseproof paper for the top of the pudding, and place on top. Wrap some foil over that, making a pleat in the middle to allow for expansion. Tie around with some string and use some more string to make a handle.

● Place the pudding basin in a steamer over a saucepan of simmering water, cover and steam for 5–6 hours. Check the water level every now and again, topping up if necessary.

● When cool, take off the paper and replace with clean greaseproof paper. Store in a cool place for up to six months, well wrapped in greaseproof paper.

● Steam again for 1½–2 hours before serving, or reheat in the microwave, which is considerably quicker.

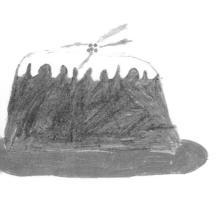

Fruity sticky toffee pudding

The sauce for this recipe contains nuts, but you can make it without if anyone has a nut allergy.

SERVES 4

225g (8oz) butter
225g (8oz) dark brown sugar
3 eggs, beaten
225g (8oz) self-raising flour
1 teaspoon baking powder
85g (3oz) stoned dates, roughly chopped
85g (3oz) dried apricots, roughly chopped
1 teaspoon bicarbonate of soda

1 teaspoon vanilla essence
300ml (10fl oz) boiling water

For the toffee walnut sauce
115g (4oz) butter
55g (2oz) dark brown sugar
4 teaspoons single cream or crème fraîche
55g (2oz) shelled walnuts, broken in half

Freeze when baked and cooled. Defrost and reheat in a low oven for 10 minutes before covering with toffee sauce and completing as given in the method.

● Preheat the oven to 180°C/350°F/Gas 4. Lightly grease a 1.2 litre (2 pint) flameproof dish.

● Cream the butter and the sugar together in a bowl until light. Gradually beat the eggs into the creamed mixture.

● Sift the flour with the baking powder. In a separate small bowl mix the dates and apricots with the bicarbonate of soda, vanilla essence, 1 tablespoon flour (taken from the measured amount) and the boiling water. Stir until well combined.

● Fold both the sifted flour and the date combination into the creamed mixture. Mix until evenly combined. Pour into the prepared dish and cook in the preheated oven for 25–30 minutes or until springy to the touch.

● Meanwhile make the toffee walnut sauce. Put the butter in a small pan and melt over a low heat. Add the sugar, bring to the boil, and then remove from the heat. Stir in the cream and walnuts and pour the sauce over the cake when it comes out of the oven.

● Put the pudding under a hot grill for a couple of minutes until the sauce bubbles. Serve with vanilla ice-cream.

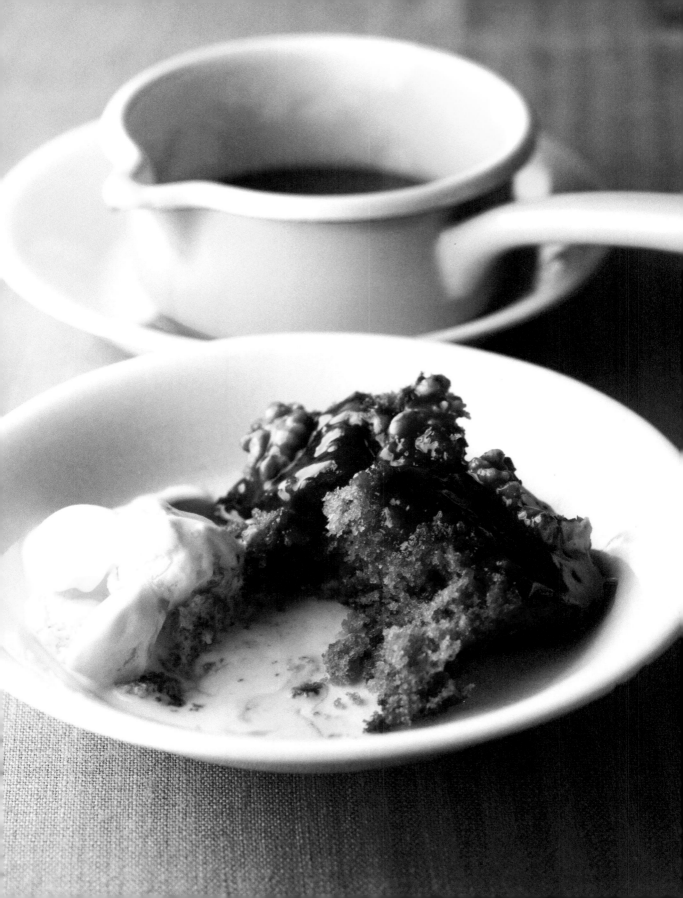

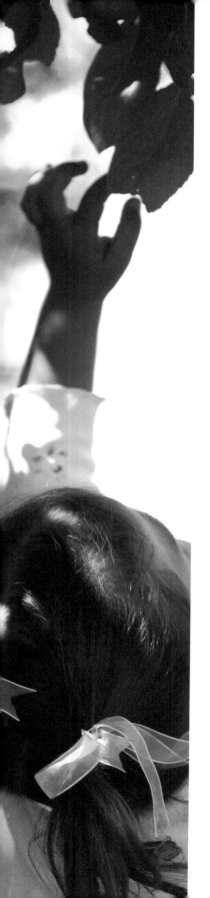

Fruit sauces

These sauces are very simple, and can make all the difference to a plain piece of sponge cake, a scoop of ice-cream or a sliced banana. They are made by puréeing fruit with a little sugar and a hint of something else, depending on the fruit. You can use raspberries, strawberries, fresh apricots, ripe kiwi fruit, plums, cherries, peaches and nectarines. If harder fruits are under-ripe, poach them a little first, in a sugar syrup. You could use canned fruit too, instead of fresh. You could even use fruit jams, although they are sometimes a bit sweet (apricot jam mixed with some fresh orange juice tastes good, and takes no time at all to make).

You can make a fruit fool by mixing a fruit sauce with thick Greek yoghurt and/or crème fraîche. You can freeze any of the sauces (in special containers or small plastic beakers with a stick) to make fruit lollies.

SERVES 4

625g (1lb 6oz) fruit
water to taste
caster sugar to taste
flavouring of choice (see below)

● Wash the fruit as appropriate, and remove any stones or pips as necessary. Put in a blender, and whiz to a purée. Push through a sieve into a bowl.

● Add water until the sauce is the consistency you want. Taste and add sugar if it is needed (this will depend on the sweetness and ripeness of the fruit). You can add another flavouring if you like (see below).

Fruit sauce flavourings

● Orange or lemon juice

● A little freshly grated nutmeg

● A little almond essence (good with peaches)

● Rosewater or orange-flower water

● A pinch of ground cinnamon

Real chocolate custard

I included the basic home-made 'real' custard recipe in my last book, and you should try it, using organic eggs and milk, as it is really creamy. You can use vanilla essence as suggested, but if you can find a vanilla pod, slice it open and use the seeds and the pod in the milk. If you want a plain custard, simply omit the cocoa powder.

SERVES 4

4 egg yolks
30g (1¼ oz) caster sugar
15g (½ oz) cornflour
a few drops pure vanilla essence
25g (1oz) cocoa powder
600ml (1 pint) milk

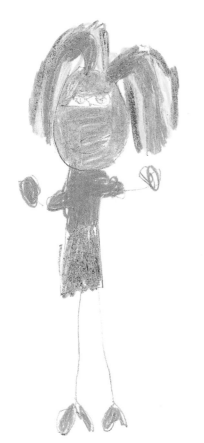

● Beat the egg yolks and sugar well, then mix in the cornflour, vanilla essence and cocoa powder.

● Bring the milk to the boil in a heavy-based saucepan. Gradually pour the hot milk into the egg yolks, whisking all the time. Return the mixture to the saucepan and heat gently over a very low heat, still whisking, until the custard thickens, about 5 minutes.

● Serve straight away.

Cakes and biscuits

Mince pies

When I went to college, which is a number of years ago now, the cookery teacher, Rae Hold, gave us a recipe for mince pies with a difference. They have cream cheese in them, and are made with orange pastry. I made them at St Peter's for the first time a few years ago, and the teachers were giving me orders for home …

MAKES 12

For the pastry
225g (8oz) self-raising flour
115g (4oz) butter, cubed
juice and rind of 1 large orange
milk to brush pastry

For the filling
115g (4oz) cream cheese
25g (1oz) icing sugar
225g (8oz) mincemeat

Freeze when cooked and reheat before serving.

● Put the flour into a large bowl and add the cubes of butter along with the orange rind. Rub the butter into the flour until the mixture resembles fine breadcrumbs. Add 2 tablespoons of the orange juice, a little at a time, bringing the mixture together with a round-ended knife. Wrap in clingfilm and place in the fridge for about 20 minutes to rest. Add the remaining orange juice to the mincemeat.

● Preheat the oven to 220°C/425°F/Gas 7. Butter some bun or muffin tins.

● In a bowl mix the cream cheese and icing sugar together. Put to one side.

● Unwrap the pastry and on a lightly floured board divide into two pieces, one piece being slightly larger. Roll out this larger piece of pastry until very thin then, using a cutter slightly larger than the diameter of your bun tins, cut out as many rounds as you need. Continue until you have filled all of the bun tins with pastry bases. Then add ½ teaspoon of the mincemeat to each, and top this with ½ teaspoon of the cream cheese mixture. Brush the edges of the pastry with water. Roll out the remaining piece of pastry to the same thickness, and, using a slightly smaller cutter, make the lids. Press these firmly on to the bases, and with a pair of scissors make a small nick to let the steam escape. Brush the tops with milk.

● Bake for 20 minutes in the preheated oven. Leave the mince pies in the tins until they are nearly cold, then lift out very carefully on to a cooling rack. Dust with extra icing sugar to serve.

271

Cut-and-come-again cake

This cake could also be served as a pudding, with a mixture of berries or a fruit salad.

MAKES 1 CAKE

225g (8oz) butter, softened, plus
    extra for greasing cake tin
225g (8oz) caster sugar
4 eggs, beaten
finely grated rind of 1 lemon
1 teaspoon vanilla essence
300g (10½ oz) self-raising flour
1 teaspoon baking powder
1 teaspoon bicarbonate of soda
225g (8oz) plain live bio-yoghurt

For the lemon syrup
115g (4oz) caster sugar
juice and thinly pared rind of
    1 lemon

For the icing (optional)
icing sugar
lemon juice

❄
Freeze when cooked,
and thaw before
decorating.

● Preheat the oven to 180°F/350°F/Gas 4. Grease and line the base of a deep 25cm (10in) cake tin or a 1.3 litre (2¼ pint) terrine tin.

● Cream the butter and caster sugar together in a bowl until smooth and the mixture turns pale. Gradually beat the eggs into the creamed mixture. Add the lemon rind and vanilla essence.

● Sift together the flour, baking powder and bicarbonate of soda. Fold half the flour into the creamed mixture, then fold in the yoghurt, followed by the remaining flour. The batter should have a dropping consistency. Spoon into the baking tin. Bake in the preheated oven for about 45–50 minutes, or until springy to the touch.

● Meanwhile make the lemon syrup. Heat the sugar with the lemon juice until the sugar dissolves, then add the lemon rind and bubble the mixture for 5 minutes. Remove the poached lemon rind and set aside for decoration.

● Remove the cake from the oven. While the cake is still warm and in its tin, drizzle the syrup over it. Set aside to cool before turning out and decorating.

● For the icing, if using, gradually mix the icing sugar with the lemon juice until it comes together as a smooth, thin icing. Drizzle the icing over the cake and decorate with the poached lemon rind pieces.